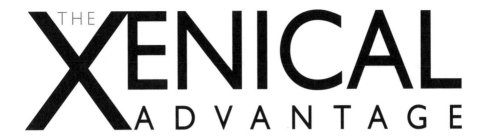

THE XENICAL ADVANTAGE

How to Use the Remarkable New FDA-Approved Drug

to Lose Weight Faster—and Keep It Off—

Safely and Effectively

John P. Foreyt, Ph.D.

with

Kristine M. Napier, M.P.H., R.D.

Illustrations by Michael J. Brown

Produced by The Philip Lief Group, Inc.

SIMON & SCHUSTER

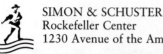

SIMON & SCHUSTER
Rockefeller Center
1230 Avenue of the Americas, New York, NY 10020

Recipes for The Moistest Pumpkin Muffins, Kris's Split Pea Soup, and Totally Decadent
Banana Chocolate Chip Muffins from *Eat to Heal* by Kristine Napier. Copyright ©
1998 by Kristine M. Napier, M.P.H., R.D. By permission of Warner Books, Inc.

Recipes for The Moistest Pumpkin Muffins, Creamed Chicken on Toast (adapted),
Creamy Breakfast Barley with Bananas and Dried Cranberries, Favorite Tuna Pasta
Salad, Vegetable Lentil Soup (adapted), Italian Chicken and Rice, One Pot Chili, and
Chicken and Zucchini Spaghetti from *Power Nutrition for Your Chronic Illness* by Kristine M. Napier. Copyright © 1998 by Kristine Napier, M.P.H., R.D. By permission of
Macmillan Books.

Recipes for Shrimp Slaw with Jicama, Pineapple and Watercress; Penne with Grilled
Chicken and Forest Mushrooms; Herb-Seared Day Boat Cod with Fresh Stewed
Tomatoes; Breast of Chicken with Braised White Beans and Arugula; Parsnip Whipped
Potatoes; Grilled Asparagus and Leeks; Old-Fashioned Apple and Fresh Raspberry
Cobbler; Peach Creamsicle Sundae with Marion Blackberry Fruit Perfect; and Warm
Pear and Blueberry Granola Crisp with Maple Yogurt by Larry P. Forgione, chef and
proprietor of An American Place, Rose Hill, and The Coach House in New York City,
and The Beekman 1766 Tavern at the Beekman Arms in Rhinebeck, New York.

All remaining recipes by Kristine M. Napier, M.P.H., R.D.

Height/weight tables adapted from 1983 Metropolitan Life Insurance Company
height/weight table, reprinted with permission, *Statistical Bulletin*, 1983.

BMI table adapted from National Heart, Lung and Blood Institute.

Xenical is a registered trademark of Hoffmann-LaRoche. This book is not affiliated
with or authorized or endorsed by Hoffmann-LaRoche, the manufacturer of Xenical.

Designed by Pagesetters, Inc.
Manufactured in the United States of America

10   9   8   7   6   5   4   3   2   1

Library of Congress Cataloging-in-Publication Data is available.

ISBN 0-684-83978-4

Note to Readers
This publication contains the opinions and ideas of its author. It is intended to provide
helpful and informative material on the subjects addressed in the publication. It is sold
with the understanding that the author and publisher are not engaged in rendering medical, health, or any other kind of personal or professional services in the book. The
reader should consult his or her medical, health, or other competent professional before
adopting any of the suggestions in this book or drawing inferences from it.

The author and the publisher specifically disclaim all responsibility for any liability,
loss, or risk, personal or otherwise, that is incurred as a consequence, directly or indirectly, of the use and application of any of the contents of this book.

Acknowledgments

The Xenical Advantage could not have been written without the help, dedication, and support of many colleagues. I especially want to thank my coauthor, Kristine Napier, who put her life on hold to work on this book with me. Kris understands the challenges experienced by those individuals who struggle constantly with their weight and try to develop or maintain a healthy lifestyle. She is a terrific writer and is able to convey clearly the steps involved in changing one's life. Kris was the key to writing the book on time and in a form we are both proud of. She also developed and tested all her heart-healthy meal plans, menus, and recipes. I feel a deep sense of gratitude and owe many thanks to Kris.

I want to thank Fiona Hinton and Judy Linden at the Philip Lief Group for their never-ending enthusiasm, encouragement, and great editorial skills in guiding the book from its initial conception to completion. Fiona and Judy were always available to share their expertise and make sure that this book became a reality. Thanks to Bob Bender, Johanna Li, Aileen Boyle, and colleagues at Simon & Schuster who provided encouragement and constant support.

My special appreciation goes to the professionals at Roche Laboratories, especially Charles P. Lucas, Gary Nichols, Thomas Klein, Jonathan Hauptman, Russell Ellison, Philippe Burnham, Karen Segal, Jean C. Burge, Francis J. Peterson, Dennis W. Joubert, Valerie Suga, Alexander Danyluk, and Geraldine D. Anastasio, who were available at all times to answer questions about Xenical. Roche Laboratories also funded our research studies on Xenical, and I am deeply grateful for their support. The Roche representatives and other Roche professionals whom I have met and worked closely with over the years have helped me focus this book. Among them I especially want to thank Mark Orth, Cecil Fuselier, V. Denise Gray, Tal Gardenhire, Vanda Gill, Bill Sullivan, Ken Thomas, Kuulei Alama-Francis, Brian Bogenschutz, Jerry McCarthy, John Herbst, Lauri Littlewood, Caroline Becker, Cliff Stagg, Brad Deslatte, Jay Briggs, Craig Schwemin, Suzanne Faubel, Willie Polk, Cathy Pedulla, and Katharine E. Marshall for their help and friendship. Special thanks to Frederique Welgryn, Jean-Michel Joubert, Monelle

Muntlak, and Didier Laloye from Roche France; Valerie Ede from Roche Brazil; Sharon Williams from Roche Australia; Robin Van from Roche Canada; Franciosa Briones from Roche Philippines; and Miroslava Santander, Armando Ramirez, and Monica Saldivar from Roche Mexico. Kiersten Rogers, Harry Wade, and Christine Landy at Stratis KPR provided background information and support for this endeavor.

My gratitude goes to Larry Forgione, well-known New York chef and restaurant proprietor, for his contribution of some delicious recipes.

I am indebted to my good friend and colleague Louis Aronne, M.D., for contributing the excellent foreword to the book. Lou is one of the leading obesity researchers and clinicians in this country, and I appreciate his taking the time from his hectic schedule to contribute.

My colleagues at the Baylor Behavioral Medicine Research Center— Rebecca Reeves, Carlos Poston, Pat Pace, Ken Goodrick, Devin Volding, and Dora Delgado—carried my workload to let me write this book, and I thank them for it. I could not have finished it without their help.

All the researchers on Xenical worldwide were instrumental in the preparation of this book. Their studies demonstrated the drug's safety and efficacy and showed how Xenical can make a major difference in the lives of many indivudals who have struggled with their weight. I especially appreciate my friend Steven B. Heymsfield's support.

Finally, and most important, I want to thank the thousands of patients I have worked with over the past twenty-five years. Their struggles, honesty, friendship, and courage have been a constant inspiration to me, and I dedicate this book to them.

Contents

Foreword   9

Introduction

A Brand-New Look at an Age-Old Health Concern   11

The Problem • The Solution

Chapter 1

Xenical: History, Highlights, and How Xenical Can Help You   17

What Is Xenical? • From Europe to the United States: A Brief History • Scientific Spotlight: Clinical Trials and Triumphs • Safety Evidence from Around the World • How Xenical Speeds Weight Loss • Why Xenical Is Different from Every Other Diet Drug • Other Health Benefits of Xenical • Conclusion—and a New Era

Chapter 2

How to Take Xenical for Optimal Effects   30

Beyond the Bathroom Scale: Is Xenical Right for You? • Issues to Discuss with Your Doctor • The Principles of the Xenical Program • Taking Xenical Properly • The Xenical Diet and Exercise Program: An Overview • Using Xenical with Other Diets

Chapter 3

Dieting with Xenical: The Principles   47

Food and the Head • Food Is More than Calories: Understanding Food • Can Margaret Lose Weight on 1,500 Calories? • Watch What You Eat • Xenical: Tipping the Scales in Your Favor

Chapter 4

Our Menus and Recipes 69

First Things First: Common Concerns and Fast Facts • How to Use Our Menus • Controlling Portion Sizes: Tips and Hints • Menus • Recipes

Chapter 5

On Your Own: Creating Your Own Menus and Eating Out 141

What Is in a Serving? • Keeping Records: Your Personal Food Diary • Monitoring Fat: Guidelines and Tables • Into the Kitchen: Two More Strategies • The Real World: Eating Out • What If I'm Tempted to Eat a Very High-Fat Food?

Chapter 6

Exercising with Xenical: Designing Your Individual Fat-Burning Program 156

About Our Exercise Program • Choose Critically: Love How You Move • How Much You Should Exercise • Top Ten Fat-Burning Exercises • Exercise Program Number One: Walking • Exercise Program Number Two: Cross-Training • Weight Training: Help Your Body Help You Lose Weight • The Exercise Advantage

Chapter 7

I've Hit My Goal Weight! Now What? 179

Should You Keep Taking Xenical? • The Weight-Maintenance Diet • The Xenical Weight-Maintenance Program • Recipes • The Maintenance Program on Your Own • Keeping Records—Your Personal Food Diary • How to Avoid Gaining Back Lost Weight

Chapter 8

Safety Concerns 221

When You Should Not Take Xenical • When to Use Xenical Cautiously (or Maybe Not at All) • Taking Xenical Correctly • About Fat-Soluble Vitamins • About Breast Cancer and Xenical • Overall Safety

References 229

Index 235

Foreword

Over the last decade, the epidemic of overweight and obesity has captured national attention in medical circles as well as the media. This problem, which afflicts over half the adult U.S. population and a growing number of children, appears to be simple to solve but is, in fact, frustratingly difficult to treat. If people would just maintain a nutritious, low-calorie diet and do regular exercise, we are told, many of their health problems, from excess body weight to heart disease to adult-onset diabetes, would disappear. Unfortunately, several factors make this advice difficult to follow. Once excess weight is gained, the body does not want to give it up. In the past this served an important purpose, for body fat is an efficient way of storing calories for later use, kind of like carrying a refrigerator around with you. Our ancestors developed these mechanisms to protect them from starving to death during times of famine. Fortunately, we now live in a land of plenty, but these adaptations to life in the wild have become maladaptive and have saddled us with the burden of obesity.

In order to lose weight, you need to know what to eat, what makes a healthy diet. But perhaps more important, you need to be able to comply with this advice, for even when you are equipped with this knowledge, weight loss is a long, difficult road with many setbacks thanks to these survival mechanisms. As anyone who has struggled with his or her weight knows, there is a world of difference between knowing what to do and doing it.

Many people in the United States are searching for a solution to their weight problem, looking for anything that can lend them a helping hand in their quest to lose weight and be healthier. Doctors, too, have now begun to realize that some people are simply not able to lose weight on their own. Until recently the only medicinal help came from appetite suppressants that were approved for short-term use. The entire category of drugs was regarded with concern when Redux, a popular appetite suppressant, was withdrawn from the market because of side effects. Last year a new medication, Meridia, became available as the first centrally acting medication (meaning that it acts in the brain) approved for long-term use. Although Meridia has helped many people succeed, no medication works well for everyone. Some people have contraindications to its use, do not respond to its effect, or have side effects.

We now have a new FDA-approved medication to offer hope to those at war with their weight. Xenical is the first prescription medication that helps people lose weight by reducing the body's absorption of dietary fat. This drug, which has been studied by researchers around the world for periods as long as two years, works in a way unlike any weight-control medication that has come before it. Because it acts in the digestive tract to reduce fat absorption and is minimally absorbed into the bloodstream, Xenical does not appear to cause the systemic side effects seen with other weight-control medications. In addition, Xenical reinforces compliance with a healthy, low-fat diet because its gastrointestinal side effects, such as fecal urgency and oily stools, generally occur only if someone eats too much fat. Xenical is not the magic bullet that everyone dreams of whereby all weight problems would be solved by just popping a pill. Any drug which makes that promise is literally too good to be true!

Remember, not only do you need to know what to eat to lose weight and be healthy, but you must also have all the behavioral resources necessary to help you comply with those recommendations. This applies whether or not you're taking Xenical. That's where *The Xenical Advantage* comes in. In addition to explaining how Xenical works and how to take it for optimal results, Dr. John Foreyt details a diet that he has tailored especially for use with Xenical. And because John's specialty is behavioral strategies for weight control, he is the ideal person to provide tools to help people with the difficult side of the equation—sticking with the diet. This "user's guide" also covers other important details pertaining to Xenical therapy, from the issues they should discuss with their doctor when deciding whether this medication is right for them to an exercise plan that will help them improve their fitness and maintain their lost weight. In an ideal world, everyone would be able to lose and maintain lost weight without the need for medications such as Xenical. In the real world, however, some people need and will benefit from the help that weight-control medications can provide. If a medication can safely give people the impetus they need to lose their excess pounds and improve their health, I'm in favor of it. If, like Xenical, it can reinforce a healthy diet that can also reduce the risk of problems such as diabetes and heart disease, then so much the better. If you are thinking about taking Xenical, I urge you to learn to use it appropriately, and for that I recommend that you read *The Xenical Advantage*.

Louis J. Aronne, M.D., F.A.C.P.
Clinical Associate Professor of Medicine
Weill Medical College of Cornell University
Director, Comprehensive Weight Control Program

A Brand-New Look at an Age-Old Health Concern

I have been helping men and women lose weight for over twenty-five years and so am intimately acquainted with the difficult struggle it entails. I have watched thousands of people battle yo-yo dieting—losing, regaining, and repeating the cycle many times over. I know these people are sincere, that they really are trying to slim down. I also know that many overweight people focus their lives, year after year, on this one task.

Cindy, a thirty-four-year-old bank customer service manager from Houston, represents thousands of these people who so desperately want to lose weight and who have tried every weight-loss trick and gimmick that has come along. "I was always a chunky child but really blew up after the birth of my child in 1990," says Cindy. For the next three years, Cindy tried everything. She tried every type of 1,000-calorie—starvation—diet she could find. "But every one of those diets failed. I would lose quickly but then gain back the weight just as fast. I was constantly hungry on them."

Then Cindy was asked to try Xenical in one of the medication's first clinical trials. "When they told me I could eat 1,500 calories and lose weight, I was skeptical. I had always associated diets with deprivation," says Cindy. But she was soon pleasantly surprised. The weight started coming off—steadily. After one year of taking Xenical and following the prescribed diet and exercise plan, Cindy dropped 35 pounds, plummeting from 201 pounds to 166. In the second year she lost another 13 pounds, reaching 153 pounds. At the end of two years Cindy stopped taking Xenical but continued the lifestyle changes she learned while on the medication—eating a fabulously healthy and reasonable calorie meal plan and exercising regularly. Four years after she stopped taking

Xenical, Cindy has gradually dropped another 23 pounds—and is confident she can maintain this 71-pound weight loss.

Xenical represents a significant breakthrough in weight control. This remarkable weapon in the battle of the bulge boasts excellent results, helping dieters lose weight at an accelerated rate as well as maintain their weight loss. Of even greater consequence, though, is how Xenical works: its unique mode of action grants it a double-pronged advantage. It both prevents dangerous side effects and helps answer every dieter's dream of maintaining weight loss. This is because Xenical is specifically designed to work by helping people change their diet to establish the healthy lifestyle necessary to live a slimmer life.

Xenical is the first of a new class of weight-control drugs that act exactly where needed: in the digestive tract. There, Xenical reduces the body's fat absorption by inhibiting the action of lipases, body chemicals that break down and facilitate the absorption of the fat in our diet. People taking Xenical absorb only about two-thirds of the fat they eat. The other third, with the associated calories, passes directly out of the body via the digestive tract. This mode of action is in sharp contrast to every other previous prescription diet drug, which were all developed to act on the brain, usually by suppressing appetite.

In fact, the way appetite suppressants work puts them at an immediate disadvantage. Because they have to be absorbed into the bloodstream and then travel to the brain, these diet drugs have the opportunity to cause side effects in other parts of the body. Indeed, some of them—Redux and Pondimin—were linked to damaged heart and lung tissue in some people who took them. The potential for serious side effects was so great that the drugs were no longer prescribed. But we also came to realize that they would never solve the weight problem of most overweight people. This is because, as appetite suppressants, they did not allow people to eat normally and never gave them the opportunity to learn to take charge of their eating habits.

In contrast, Xenical works both in the short term to accelerate weight loss but also long term to help people keep off the pounds that they already shed. Xenical also allows dieters to take charge, to establish a routine of healthy diet and exercise while taking the medication.

The Problem

Despite a seemingly bottomless well of weight-loss aids and programs, the percentage of Americans at war with their weight has reached alarming proportions. One in four American women (25 percent) and one in five American men (20 percent) are obese. Add to this the 39.4 percent of men and 24.7 percent of women who are overweight, and we find that well over half of the American population is too heavy. Startlingly, most of this increase has occurred this past decade.

Although many of the people who come to me for help are driven to diet for cosmetic reasons—fitting into last season's clothes, looking trim at the beach, and so on—the consequences of carrying around too much weight cut much deeper than the issue of appearance. I often see people whose weight problems are so severe that their very lives are in jeopardy unless they shed pounds. People with serious and life-threatening heart disease, diabetes raging out of control, and arthritis that is literally crippling them come to me for urgent answers to the weight problems that have negatively impacted their lives. It is wise to remember, however, that weight-associated health troubles begin long before people reach the official designation of obesity.

The following are among the problems suffered by those who are overweight and the reasons to make every effort to slim down to a healthier body weight:

High Blood Pressure. Carrying just twenty extra pounds raises blood pressure enough to increase the risk of heart disease by about 12 percent and the risk of stroke about 24 percent. On the other hand, losing weight is one of the most effective nonpharmacological methods of lowering blood pressure.

High Blood Cholesterol Levels. While both overweight men and women have higher cholesterol levels than their normal-weight counterparts, levels seem to climb even higher in women as they gain weight.

Atherosclerosis, or Coronary Artery Disease. The risk of artery-clogging heart disease increases at even modest levels of overweight. Weight gains of eleven to eighteen pounds over the healthy range increase a person's chance of suffering heart disease (measured as both heart attack and death from heart disease) by an astonishing 25 percent.

Diabetes Mellitus. About one in four cases of adult-onset diabetes can be traced to weight gain in the adult years; gaining just five kilograms, or eleven pounds, dramatically increases the risk.

Congestive Heart Failure. Because it is working hard to pump blood to so much extra tissue, the heart muscle of overweight people has a greater chance of wearing out or suffering congestive heart failure. When this condition advances, the only solution may be a heart transplant.

Stroke. Largely because of weight-associated increases in blood pressure, stroke risk is considerably higher in people who are overweight or obese. Compared to normal-weight women, the risk of stroke is 75 percent higher in overweight women and 137 percent higher in those who are obese.

Osteoarthritis. Simply put, the human skeleton has a weight limit. This complex system of bones and connective tissue just isn't meant to support more than a certain number of pounds. This explanation makes it easier to understand why gaining just 1 kilogram (2.2 pounds) increases the chance of developing osteoarthritis in women by 9 to 13 percent. Excess weight basically grinds away the skeletal system. In addition, weight gain is one of the main reasons that joints become painful.

Gallstones. Excess body weight increases the risk of developing gallstones in both men and women, but the increase is even more dramatic in women. While about 9.4 percent of normal-weight women suffer from gallstones, 25.5 percent of obese women do.

Cancer. Studies suggest that obesity may double the risk of colon cancer and that it increases the death rate from breast cancer in post-menopausal women. Obesity triples the risk of endometrial cancer in women.

Depression: Obesity represents a risk factor for depression.

(Scientists studying Xenical have shown that, in concert with increased rates of weight loss, this medication effectively reduces several of these health risks, including blood pressure, cholesterol levels, and diabetes indicators.)

Compared to the often serious health problems associated with obesity, the cosmetic issues seem trivial. Indeed, if it were only about looks, there wouldn't be such an urgency to find ways to help the one in two overweight Americans lose weight and keep it off. But given the potentially momentous aftermath of gaining weight, we are desperate to find more effective ways to facilitate weight loss.

The Solution

As a weight-loss expert, I know that in order to succeed at living a healthier life, a person ultimately must refashion his or her lifestyle, exercising regularly and eating a sensible diet. This is where I assist people in becoming aware of their eating habits, understanding what makes them eat, and then identifying how to change these habits to a style that gradually leads to and then helps them maintain a healthier weight. As anyone who has tried to lose weight knows, this isn't just about knowing what to eat; it is just as much about how and when to eat.

I have been involved with the weight wars long enough and intimately enough to know that not everyone can win the battle alone. It is clear that certain people need help in their efforts; they need a little assistance down the road to a slimmer life. This is where a medication such as Xenical comes in. In addition to boosting your rate of weight loss, it allows you to learn to take control of your eating habits, to make the transition to a new lifestyle.

As with any medication, though, Xenical will be effective only if used properly—in the context of an appropriate diet and exercise program, as intended by its developers. By following the guidelines presented in this book, you can maximize Xenical's benefits and your weight loss.

In *The Xenical Advantage* you will learn about:

- Xenical's twenty-five-year history and research highlights detailing its effectiveness;
- how Xenical speeds weight loss;
- the optimal use of Xenical;
- what and how you should eat to maximize Xenical's benefits;
- the behavioral strategies that complement your weight-loss efforts and, more important, that you need to observe to maintain your weight-loss achievements;
- the diet plans necessary to maintain weight loss after Xenical;
- exercise programs that are essential to speeding and maintaining weight loss;
- vitamin supplements needed when taking Xenical and how to take them;
- how to use Xenical in conjunction with other weight-loss programs, including Weight Watcher's and Jenny Craig;
- what to do when you've reached your weight goal.

Most importantly, we discuss essential safety information for anyone considering using Xenical. Chapter 8, Safety Concerns, covers the potential drug interactions and contraindications that may occur with this medication. For example, if you take warfarin, a blood thinner, or pravastatin, a cholesterol-lowering drug, you may not be a candidate for Xenical. Also, you should not take Xenical if you are under eighteen or over sixty-five, or if you have chronic malabsorption, which means that your gastrointestinal tract does not absorb nutrients as well as it should. This may occur if you have Crohn's disease or if you have had some of your bowel surgically removed.

My mission is to help you win at the weight-loss game. By using Xenical in conjunction with the specially tailored diet and exercise information in *The Xenical Advantage,* you can make the transition to a healthier, slimmer life once and for all.

1

Xenical: History, Highlights, and How
Xenical Can Help You

What Is Xenical?

Xenical is the first of a new class of weight-loss drugs called lipase inhibitors that act by reducing the body's absorption of fat. Xenical is the trade name and orlistat is the chemical name for the only prescription drug of this kind that is available around the world. A welcome innovation, Xenical is the product of a quarter-century of research to find an effective weight-loss drug.

From Europe to the United States: A Brief History

In the 1970s, obesity researchers first contemplated the preferred action of an effective weight-loss drug. Prior to this, the only experience had been with amphetamines, which were prescribed to suppress appetite but were soon found to have many undesirable and even dangerous side effects. Pharmaceutical researchers at Hoffmann-LaRoche's laboratories in Nutley, New Jersey, began the search for a drug that would have a very focused target of action, hoping to eliminate the side effects problem. They decided to try to develop a drug that would act directly in the intestinal tract to block the absorption of fat in that area, and soon started looking for the optimal pancreatic lipase inhibitor.

Here is why their search makes sense scientifically. Pancreatic lipases are the enzymes, or chemical knives, that break apart dietary fat into its constituent parts, into a size the body can absorb. Finding the right drug to stop the action of lipase would possibly mean that fat would remain in larger-sized chains that would be too large to be assimilated into the cells of the intestinal tract. In turn, the researchers hoped, some of the dietary fat would pass out of the body unabsorbed.

Why target dietary fat? For several reasons. First, while we do need some dietary fat to live, we need small amounts—much less than we take in. Americans, for example, eat an average of 78 grams of fat daily. To meet the body's need for fat (which it uses to make hormones and tissue membranes and to absorb fat-soluble vitamins, for example), we require around 20 grams daily. So getting rid of some of the dietary fat we eat isn't harmful.

Another reason to target dietary fat with a weight-loss drug is that fat is the most calorically dense macronutrient we eat. Three types of nutrients, called macronutrients, supply the body with the energy it needs to keep going: carbohydrates, protein, and fat. Both carbohydrates and protein supply approximately 4 calories per gram (the actual value ranges from 3.8 to 4.1). As a means of understanding how big a gram is, note that there are about 28 grams per ounce; a prewrapped slice of cheese, for example, weighs approximately one ounce. Fats, on the other hand, are two and one-quarter times as calorically dense as carbohydrates and protein, supplying about 9 calories per gram.

Because of the calorie content of fats, it is very easy to take in a significant number of fat calories quickly. Worse yet, fat is not necessarily the most appetite-squelching macronutrient. According to some researchers, it is the volume of food we eat that leads to the feeling of satiety that makes us stop eating. This is why some people find it so easy to down a piece of fat-laden chocolate cheese cake but difficult to finish a large but calorie-light salad.

In the 1970s search for the best lipase inhibitor, Roche researchers had no fewer than 1,000 candidates. Although about one-fifth of them showed some promise in test-tube research, none affected body weight when tested in animals. To facilitate their search, researchers joined forces with the Roche research team in Basel, Switzerland, which had developed a screening test that accelerated the search, allowing scientists to test up to 150 substances per week. Between 1977 and 1981 alone, the investigators tested 5,000 lipase inhibitors in rats and 10,000 in mice.

Finally, one substance showed true promise. It was the first that hooked up with pancreatic lipases and stopped them from breaking fat molecules into pieces small enough for the body to absorb. The effect, however, was too short-lived to help. The lipases broke away from the inhibitor and still digested fat molecules, allowing all the dietary fat to be absorbed.

In their next phase of research, investigators turned to bacteria and fungi, prolific producers of biologically active proteins. Several teams of researchers joined together, trying to find the bacteria that produced a protein molecule that would irreversibly stop pancreatic lipases. Some scientists, bent on their quest, even worked while vacationing. It was a Roche scientist on holiday in Majorca, Spain, who finally found the best bacterium. On a whim, he collected a soil sample from the beach where he should have been sunning and relaxing, and sent it back to his laboratory for analysis. Serendipitously, it was that sample that contained the long-sought bacterium: *Streptomyces toxitricini*. This one bacteria came from testing more than fifteen thousand substances in a total of 3,165 different culture mediums ("broths").

The process was fascinating but tedious. Scientists knew *S. toxitricini* produced the molecule for which they were searching, but they soon discovered that this "holy grail" molecule was fragile. They had to extract the active molecule from the broth by dividing the broth into chemically different fractions and then testing each fraction for lipase inhibitory activity. However, the molecule was so fragile that the purification process destroyed it. Fortunately, researchers figured out a way around this glitch, designing a new purification process that did not break up the molecule. The scientists were ecstatic, having achieved the first major step toward success.

The next step was to figure out what made the molecule work— knowledge that would allow scientists to understand the substance and then reproduce it in large quantities if it still proved effective. This involved structural analysis, or tearing down the molecule bit by bit to identify its building blocks and how they were pieced together.

In October 1982 scientists identified the chemical nature of the active substance and named it "lipstatin," from the word parts "lipo" meaning fat and "statin" meaning "to stop." Further work revealed that lipstatin did not hold up at room temperature. But scientists soon solved this problem by adding four molecules of hydrogen to the formula, which stabilized it at room temperature. The new compound was named tetrahydrolipstatin, from the word parts "tetra" for four and "hydro" for hydrogen. Because tetrahydrolipstatin was such a mouthful, scientists gave it another name: orlistat.

Over the next five years the pharmaceutical researchers answered important questions and solved problems. They assessed orlistat's safety, deciding it appeared safe and lacked toxicity. Most important, they wanted to make sure that orlistat did not leave the intestinal tract and enter the bloodstream. They knew this was key in preventing side effects in other parts of the body. They also wanted to be certain that orlistat did not harm the cells in the intestinal tract in the process of blocking fat absorption. This, too, was critical in establishing safety. Their testing and retesting were rewarded positively: all tests showed that less than 1 percent of orlistat was absorbed and that it was not toxic to intestinal cells.

After determining its safety, orlistat researchers went back to verify the drug's ability to limit the amount of dietary fat absorbed. They weren't content to know that orlistat worked in some way to limit fat absorption; they needed to know that it would limit just the right amount of dietary fat. After all, the human body needs dietary fat to function properly, and scientists did not want the drug to work too well. Testing was again rewarded with the finding that orlistat would stop about one-third of dietary fat from being absorbed. Just to be sure, scientists ran the tests again and again. Their findings held solid.

Now it was time to figure out a cost-effective way to make large quantities of orlistat. This task proved as difficult as had each previous step. There could be no sacrificing quality or results. Trial and error and many months of research finally produced a top-quality method of manufacturing large quantities of orlistat in a manner that would make it affordable to the people who need to take it. This process involved cultivating *S. toxitricini* in a large enough volume to allow isolation of the active substance.

Scientific Spotlight: Clinical Trials and Triumphs

The first human trials of orlistat began in Basel, Switzerland, in 1987; they were to demonstrate that the drug worked as intended to limit intestinal fat absorption. In 1988 clinical trials were added in North America and Europe, about the time orlistat was given its current trade name of Xenical.

Overall, seven one- and two-year double-blind, placebo-controlled and randomized clinical trials involving more than four thousand people worldwide have been conducted on Xenical. In all studies, people who took Xenical with reduced calorie meals containing no more than 30 percent fat achieved faster weight loss than people in the studies who followed the same diet but took a placebo, or a sugar pill that looked and tasted like Xenical. Pooling all the data from the seven trials of Xenical show consistently excellent results, specifically:

- Almost three times as many people taking Xenical in addition to a reduced-calorie diet, as opposed to a reduced-calorie diet alone, achieved weight loss of more than 10 percent of their body weight.
- Twice as many people on Xenical lost at least 5 percent of their body weight. This is extremely significant. We know that people who lose any weight at all often have significant improvements in the measures of chronic disease risk. Losing 5 to 10 percent of body weight, for example, frequently lowers blood pressure and blood cholesterol levels. That is why you should take heart—and pride— in losing any weight at all.
- People taking Xenical lost 50 percent more weight than those on a reduced-calorie diet alone.
- People losing weight with Xenical showed measurable improvements in total and low-density lipoproteins (LDL), cholesterol (the bad cholesterol that deposits in and blocks arteries, possibly causing chest pain, heart attack, and/or stroke), and blood pressure, as well as improved blood levels of fasting glucose and insulin (these are indicators of diabetes).

What's in a Name?

Xenical has been studied in seven double-blind, placebo-controlled, and randomized clinical trials. Double-blind, placebo-controlled, and randomized clinical trials are the premier type of clinical study; their results are well respected. Placebo-controlled means that part of the study population received the real diet pill, and the other part a placebo, or a sugar pill that looks and tastes like the real thing. Double-blind means that both study participants and the medical personnel running the trials did not know which treatment the participant received, the real diet pill or the placebo. Finally, randomized means that study participants were assigned to the real diet pill group or the placebo group by a totally chance process, basically a lottery system. These precautions ensure that the study results are subjected to as little bias as possible, on the part of both the participants and the researchers.

I was one of the primary investigators on the most important study on Xenical, the results of which were published in the January 20, 1999, issue of the *Journal of the American Medical Association (JAMA)*. This study is noteworthy for several reasons. First, it was the largest double-blind, placebo-controlled, and randomized study ever designed to evaluate a diet drug therapy for weight loss and prevention of weight gain in overweight people. Second, this was the first study of any diet drug to be published in the esteemed *Journal of the American Medical Association*. It was also a long study, lasting two years.

Many weight-loss experts from around the country—in eighteen U.S. weight-loss centers, to be exact—worked together on this important research study. Like myself, other weight-loss experts want to be certain that a weight-loss aid is not only effective but exceptionally safe. That is why it was necessary to enlist the help of such a large group of people. The more people we study, the greater chance we have to detect side effects. Altogether 892 people were included in the experimental and placebo groups for the study, all of whom met the official medical criteria for obesity, which meant they had a body mass index (BMI) of at least 30 kg/m². (Chapter 2 explains this measurement and discusses the body mass index in more detail; it is one tool by which physicians assess whether or not a person is overweight, and it also helps classify the degree of overweight and the associated medical risks.) Prior to starting the study, all the participants were placed on equal footing in what is called the lead-in period. During this pre-study time, everyone is instructed in and asked to follow the diet they must adhere to during the study. In this case, it was a 30 percent meal plan containing a reduced number of calories (about 500 to 700 calories less than the participants' typical daily intake). This pre-study lead-in is important because it ensures that people understand what they must do during the study. It also helps improve compliance, or the ability to adhere to the diet, during the study.

During the first year of our study, people were randomly divided into two groups. The 668 in one group, called the intervention group, were given 120 milligrams of Xenical three times daily (one 120-milligram pill with each meal) and were asked to eat a reduced-calorie meal plan containing approximately 30 percent fat. People in the placebo group, a total of 224, were asked to follow the same diet but were given sugar pills instead of Xenical to take with each meal. Neither the participants nor the medical personnel supervising the study knew which pills were placebos and which were the real thing (which, as described earlier, made it a double-blind study).

In the second year of the study, the people in the Xenical group were subdivided into three groups: one-third continued to receive 120 milligrams of Xenical three times daily, one pill with each meal; one-third were given 60 milligrams Xenical with each meal; and one-third received a placebo with each meal.

Some of the highlights of this study include the following:

- About 4 of 10 people taking Xenical (or about 38.9 percent) along with eating a moderately reduced calorie diet lost 10 percent or more of body weight compared to just about 2.5 of 10 people on a placebo (24.6 percent) with the same moderately reduced calorie diet. That is, people in the Xenical group lost an average of 19.3 pounds, while those taking the placebo lost an average of 12.8 pounds during the first year.
- Nearly twice as many people on Xenical lost at least 5 percent of body weight compared to those taking a placebo. As said earlier, even small decreases in weight make a positive impact on measures of health. For some people it is easier to concentrate on dropping small amounts of weight, stabilizing, and then trying to lose more weight later on. This is effective, so look on it positively.
- Those who continued to take Xenical in the second year, when many participants were on a more liberal weight-maintenance diet, regained less weight during that year than those who did not, and people who took the larger dose of Xenical during the second year gained less weight than those who took the smaller dose.
- The Xenical group also benefitted in another way: they showed significant improvements in tests that measure a person's risk of heart disease and diabetes. In particular, there were statistically significant improvements in LDL cholesterol and blood insulin levels over those in the placebo group.

The overall incidence of side effects was about the same in both the placebo and Xenical groups. People who took Xenical did have more instances of gastrointestinal discomfort. The researchers are quick to point out that most of these occurred early in the study and mostly when participants ate too much fat. This is because eating more fat than is recommended means that there is a greater "dose" of unabsorbed fat to excrete, resulting in the symptoms.

Safety Evidence from Around the World

Xenical is approved by the U.S. Food and Drug Administration for use in treating obesity. Hoffman-LaRoche first submitted a New Drug Application (NDA) for Xenical to the FDA in November 1996 and received accelerated review status. By May 1997 the FDA's Endocrino-logic and Metabolic Advisory Committee unanimously recommended approval of Xenical. The unanimous vote came following a compre-hensive presentation of Xenical's clinical data regarding safety and efficacy.

But in August 1997, Roche withdrew the NDA to study a particular finding. There was an imbalance in the number of breast cancers observed between the treatment and placebo groups in the clinical tri-als. A comprehensive review of the study data found that the extra cases of breast cancer had nothing to do with the Xenical (see chapter 8 for more details) but were simply a matter of chance. So in November 1997, Roche resubmitted its NDA with analyses of the breast cancer data. Based on this scientific evidence, Roche doesn't believe that Xenical is an initiator or stimulator of breast cancer or tumors associated with breast cancer. Xenical's NDA again received accelerated review status from the FDA.

On May 12, 1998, the FDA granted approval status to Xenical, pend-ing submission of follow-up safety data from Xenical's ongoing clinical studies and agreement on final labeling. Final and full approval came April 26, 1999.

Used Around the World

Even before Xenical was approved by the FDA, it was available for use in seventeen countries around the world: Argentina, Austria, Belgium, Brazil, Chile, Denmark, Fin-land, France, Germany, Italy, Mexico, the Netherlands, New Zealand, Spain, Switzerland, Venezuela, and the United Kingdom. At the time of writing, well over a million people across the globe have taken Xenical to help their weight-loss efforts.

How Xenical Speeds Weight Loss

As briefly described earlier in this chapter, Xenical is a lipase-inhibiting drug. To understand fully how it works, let's first review how fat is absorbed in the intestinal tract.

All the macronutrients in the food we eat (carbohydrates, protein, and fat) are made of smaller building blocks joined together by chemi-cal bonds. Protein, for example, is made up of amino acids, joined together by bonds. Fat is made up of many small fat units, called triglycerides, joined together by another type of bond. Each of the macronutrient "chains" must be broken down into smaller building blocks so the body can absorb and use them. Enzymes are critical to this process; as we said earlier, they are the chemical knives that cut apart the bonds holding macronutrient chains together.

The pancreas, an organ in the abdominal cavity, makes the enzymes that break fat apart—the pancreatic lipases. Xenical is designed to lock onto the lipases. Once it has locked on, the enzyme cannot perform its job of cutting apart fat.

If you're thinking that a drug which blocks all fat absorption is dangerous, you're right. After all, the body does need some fat for good health. But Xenical doesn't work by blocking all dietary fat. The pharmaceutical researchers who developed and tested Xenical determined the dose that would block only about one-third of dietary fat from being digested and therefore from being absorbed. The other two-thirds gets broken down and absorbed as usual, ensuring that the body gets all the fat it needs for good health.

Let's examine the criteria on this in order to paint a very clear picture of why inhibiting fat digestion and absorption speeds weight loss. A person who wants to lose weight must first determine an optimal calorie level to do so. For example, an appropriate calorie level for a forty-five-year-old woman who is five feet two inches tall that will allow her to lose weight slowly (the best way to keep it off, as we'll discuss in chapter 3) is about 1,500 calories. Health experts recommend limiting fat intake to no more than 30 percent of calories, which is also the recommendation for Xenical users. For someone eating 1,500 calories, that means 450 fat calories, or 50 grams of fat per day (since each gram of fat has about 9 calories). If you add Xenical to this weight-loss plan, then 30 percent of the fat grams—and therefore 30 percent of the fat calories—will pass from the body unabsorbed. In this case, that translates into a deficit of about 135 calories from Xenical alone each day.

Over time, a daily 135-calorie deficit makes a huge difference. Here's why. To lose a pound of body weight, you have to have a 3,500-calorie deficit. Just from the calorie deficit created from Xenical alone (135 per day in this case), a person on a 1,500-calorie, 30 percent fat diet would lose an additional pound about every twenty-six days. That translates to about fourteen pounds more in the span of a year than without Xenical. Our hypothetical forty-five-year-old woman on 1,500 calories should lose about one pound per week via reduced calorie intake alone. Over six months she could lose about thirty-three pounds from reduced calorie intake and Xenical.

Why Xenical Is Different from Every Other Diet Drug

The other tremendous advantage of Xenical is that it works exactly where it is needed—and only there. All but a minuscule portion—over 99 percent, in fact—acts directly in the intestinal tract to halt fat breakdown and therefore fat absorption. Not even 1 percent of the drug is absorbed into the bloodstream. This is unlike other prescription diet drugs, which were designed to act on the brain, generally to reduce appetite.

The way these medications work puts them at an immediate disadvantage. The simple fact that they must be absorbed into the bloodstream and travel to and act on the brain means these other diet drugs carry a higher risk of producing side effects. Any drug that acts systemically or inside the body's metabolic machinery has the power to affect areas or organs within the body that are totally distinct from the targeted one. Such was the case of two of these diet drugs: Redux and Pondimin. Although they were intended to work only on the brain, they have been associated with damaged lung and heart tissue in some people who took them.

The risks associated with these two drugs were consequential enough to preclude their use. But a look at the bigger picture reveals that the very method by which they were intended to work could never make them the answer for most people who need help with their weight-loss efforts. Experience has taught us that artificially suppressing the appetite does not offer a long-term solution for many overweight people because appetite suppressants aid weight loss only as long as the person takes the drug. Indeed, we now know many users regained their weight once they stopped taking the drug. This is because a person does not have to learn the self-control and dietary changes necessary to follow a healthy diet for long-term success.

Xenical, however, is designed to help teach self-control and the long-term behavior modification necessary to change eating habits forever. There are two reasons for this. First, a person will not experience significant weight loss unless he or she cuts calorie intake while taking the drug. This is because the drug isn't meant as a magic bullet but as a tool to speed weight loss. People who take Xenical without reducing calorie intake will lose weight so slowly—perhaps a pound each month— that they might stop taking the drug because their efforts receive little reward.

Second, those who take Xenical must control their fat intake at meals and put extra thought into which snacks they eat. As we'll discuss in later chapters, each meal should contain no more than about 20 grams of fat. Eating more fat than that at any one time while taking Xenical can result in gastrointestinal troubles. This could include fecal urgency, or the need to use the bathroom suddenly, as well as loose, oily stools. Some people have experienced oily spotting as well.

Here is why snacks must include only foods that are low in fat. Xenical works to decrease fat absorption only at the time it is taken, and it should only be taken with meals. This means that if you eat fat-containing snacks between meals, you will absorb all of the fat they contain. Therefore, a person taking Xenical has to plan on healthy, very low fat snacks such as fruit, vegetables, and fat-free yogurt. You can also think of this as another means of modifying behavior, which takes you one step closer to long-term weight control. Add one more positive thought: this is the way that leading health organizations advise everyone to eat to reduce the risk of heart disease, cancer, osteoarthritis, and other diseases.

Other Health Benefits of Xenical

People with weight problems are at great risk of health troubles, especially heart disease and diabetes. While weight loss alone cuts the risk of these problems, clinical trials showed that Xenical-assisted weight loss reduces the risk even more.

Clinical trials demonstrated that people losing weight with Xenical achieved a significant reduction in blood pressure and LDL (bad) cholesterol levels and greater improvement in diabetic control than those on a reduced-calorie diet alone. At first glance one might think that the greater improvements in all these areas are simply due to the greater weight loss experienced by the Xenical takers. After all, the more weight a person loses, the more overall health improves. Data analysis is so sophisticated, however, that statisticians can often determine what factors contribute to the results and even how much weight these factors have in those results. This is called determining the magnitude of effect.

Through this advanced data analysis, researchers were able to determine that it wasn't just the extra weight loss alone that brought the greater improvement in blood LDL cholesterol levels. Xenical itself was somehow bringing about some of this improvement. Here's what happened.

After the lead-in period, during which both study groups followed the prescribed diet and neither group took Xenical, blood pressure and blood fat levels were found to have improved with this change in diet alone; this has also been shown in other dieting studies. After the lead-in period, people who took Xenical continued to show improvements in blood cholesterol readings during year one of the study period. However, the cholesterol levels of those who took the placebo increased steadily after the four-week lead-in period, even among those who continued to lose weight (although they lost less weight than people taking Xenical). The researchers believe that Xenical helps maintain improvements in blood cholesterol levels brought about by weight loss because it inhibits fat absorption. After all, it is a well-known fact that one of the main culprits in raising blood cholesterol levels is saturated fat in the diet, and one of the most effective ways to lower blood cholesterol is to reduce the amount of dietary fat. Dieting with Xenical basically exerts a triple—and positive—whammy on blood fat: Xenical dieters must eat less fat; thanks to Xenical they absorb even less of the fat they do eat; and they lose weight, which helps most people lower their blood cholesterol levels.

Measures of diabetic control also improved to a much greater extent among the Xenical group. People who have diabetes mellitus have abnormalities in their blood sugar metabolism. The problem centers on insulin, a hormone that basically unlocks the door for sugar in the blood to enter the body's cells where it is used for fuel, just as gas fuels a car. As necessary as insulin is, it can also be a problem. This is especially true when insulin levels become elevated, as they may do in people with diabetes mellitus. Although some people with diabetes can move the sugar into their cells simply by pumping out larger and larger quantities of insulin, this isn't healthy. These excessively high insulin levels have consequences, among them higher blood pressure and an extremely elevated risk of heart disease.

Fortunately, losing weight helps the body use insulin more efficiently; this is called increasing insulin sensitivity. The greater degree of weight loss in the Xenical group brought about quite significant improvements in insulin levels. Fasting insulin levels fell throughout the study in people who took Xenical, and the decrease was sustained for the full two years of the study. In sharp contrast, fasting insulin levels in the placebo group remained basically unchanged over the two years. So not only did the Xenical dieters lose more weight, but they improved their health in several other important areas, reducing the risk of many chronic diseases.

Conclusion—and a New Era

In a medical society that rebuilds hearts and cures cancer, we have almost come to take medical advances for granted. However, weight control, seemingly a simple issue, has proved a very difficult problem to solve. Xenical represents a significant advance in this arena. From the concept in the 1970s of a drug that would block absorption of the most calorically dense and spareable nutrient, research has led to a fully approved drug just twenty or so years later—seemingly long but truly short in the realm of medical research. I hope this new medication will provide a helping hand to the millions of people who sincerely struggle with weight loss, frustrated but determined to be healthier.

In chapter 2 we will discuss how to use Xenical properly and for optimal results.

2

How to Take Xenical for Optimal Effects

Let's face it. We are all tough on ourselves. Sometimes we wish we had a different shaped nose or perhaps thicker hair, and often we wish our body size or shape resembled the ones we see on television. Some of these things we simply can't change, nor should we want to. I'm a firm believer, after so many years of helping people address weight problems, that body image is a very significant part of dieting. In fact, too many people who are already healthfully trim work themselves into a frenzy to be thinner—too thin—just to get rid of what they perceive is an extra inch on hips or thighs.

Neither this book nor Xenical is intended for these people. Taking a drug to lose weight when weight loss isn't necessary could never be recommended. Although I am concerned about people with body image quandaries and hope they find a way to deal with and accept such issues, this book—like the decision to take Xenical—is about and intended for an entirely different group of people.

The diet and exercise plans and, most of all, the new hope that may be found through this book are for the many millions of Americans who have a genuine weight problem. Extra pounds for these people may carry a risk of or have already helped to cause serious illness, such as diabetes or heart disease. It is these people who should be searching for the ultimate answer to their weight loss woes, for a permanent way to bring their weight down to a level that is compatible with vibrant health and a satisfying, enjoyable way of life. If you are one of these people, let me help you decide whether Xenical can help you. Let's start by discussing the numbers that will help you make the decision.

Beyond the Bathroom Scale: Is Xenical Right for You?

As a weight-loss expert, I analyze more than the number on the scale to decide the severity of a person's weight problem. The four pieces of evidence that may be used are body weight, body mass index, waist circumference, and the presence of comorbid (other medical) conditions. Let's take a look at each of these.

Body Weight. Almost everyone has driven over a small country bridge with a weight limit, wondering if the bridge is strong enough to carry your passenger car. You know the limit that the bridge can hold because there is generally a well-worn sign that says "Weight Limit: XX Tons." I always use this analogy when I think of the weight any human body is meant to carry. Although we don't think of it this way, every person's body has a weight limit. Mother Nature created the bones of our skeletons with the ability to carry a limited amount of weight healthfully (just as engineers constructed small country bridges with the ability to hold a certain number of cars at any one time). Even more subtle than the weight limit on our skeletons is the weight limit on our blood vessels and tissues. The body has to make more blood vessels to feed the extra tissue added with weight gain (yes, fat tissue is living tissue that needs to be oxygenated and fed with blood). Ultimately, that puts extra strain on the heart, which then has to pump blood out to more tissues than originally intended. This means the lungs have to work harder, because they must fill the blood with the oxygen that is the basis of life. All this is related to help you understand that there is a limit to the amount of weight the human body is meant to carry and to help you appreciate the consequences of pushing this limit.

Unfortunately, though, we don't come with instructions or signs about healthy weight limits. That is why we need guidelines, and some people use weight tables as guidelines. Think of them as the signs telling us how much weight a bridge can hold. Refer to Tables 1 and 2, which have been updated to accommodate the latest knowledge about how weight affects health. Find your desirable weight, the weight at which your body is healthiest, by looking for your height. Officially speaking, we say a person is overweight when his or her weight is 20 percent or more above the ideal body weight. The distinction changes to obesity when weight creeps to more than 30 percent over the healthiest body weight.

Please note that these tables are considered old-fashioned when it comes to assessing people's weight problems. Those of us involved in weight control find that the body mass index, or BMI, is a far more powerful tool in understanding how weight impacts obesity, but many people still like to see where their weight should fall in these old-fashioned weight tables.

		TABLE 1		
		Desirable Weights for Men		
Height Without Shoes	Frame Size	Desirable Weight (Pounds)	Overweight (≥20% over Desirable Weight)	Obese (≥30% over Desirable Weight)
5'5"	Small	124–133	≥155	≥168
5'5"	Medium	130–143	≥164	≥178
5'5"	Large	138–156	≥176	≥191
5'6"	Small	128–137	≥160	≥173
5'6"	Medium	134–147	≥169	≥183
5'6"	Large	142–161	≥182	≥198
5'7"	Small	132–141	≥164	≥178
5'7"	Medium	138–152	≥174	≥189
5'7"	Large	147–156	≥188	≥204
5'8"	Small	136–145	≥169	≥183
5'8"	Medium	142–156	≥179	≥194
5'8"	Large	151–170	≥193	≥209
5'9"	Small	140–150	≥174	≥189
5'9"	Medium	146–160	≥184	≥200
5'9"	Large	155–174	≥198	≥214
5'10"	Small	144–154	≥179	≥194
5'10"	Medium	150–165	≥190	≥205
5'10"	Large	159–179	≥203	≥220
5'11"	Small	148–158	≥184	≥199
5'11"	Medium	154–170	≥194	≥211
5'11'	Large	164–184	≥209	≥226
6'0"	Small	152–162	≥188	≥204
6'0"	Medium	158–175	≥200	≥217
6'0"	Large	168–189	≥215	≥233

Height Without Shoes	Frame Size	Desirable Weight (Pounds)	Overweight (≥20% over Desirable Weight)	Obese (≥30% over Desirable Weight)
6'1"	Small	156–167	≥194	≥211
6'1"	Medium	162–180	≥205	≥222
6'1"	Large	173–194	≥221	≥239
6'2"	Small	160–171	≥199	≥216
6'2"	Medium	167–185	≥211	≥229
6'2"	Large	178–199	≥227	≥246
6'3"	Small	164–175	≥204	≥221
6'3"	Medium	172–190	≥217	≥235
6'3"	Large	182–204	≥232	≥302

Adapted from 1983 Metropolitan Life Insurance Company height/weight table, reprinted with permission, *Statistical Bulletin*, 1983.

TABLE 2
Desirable Weights for Women

Height Without Shoes	Frame Size	Desirable Weight (Pounds)	Overweight (≥20% over Desirable Weight)	Obese (≥30% over Desirable Weight)
5'0"	Small	102–110	≥127	≥138
5'0"	Medium	107–119	≥136	≥147
5'0"	Large	115–131	≥148	≥160
5'1"	Small	105–113	≥131	≥142
5'1"	Medium	110–122	≥139	≥151
5'1"	Large	118–134	≥151	≥164
5'2"	Small	108–116	≥134	≥146
5'2"	Medium	113–126	≥143	≥155
5'2"	Large	121–138	≥155	≥168
5'3"	Small	111–119	≥138	≥150
5'3"	Medium	116–130	≥148	≥160
5'3"	Large	125–142	≥160	≥173
5'4"	Small	114–123	≥142	≥153
5'4"	Medium	120–135	≥152	≥165
5'4"	Large	129–146	≥164	≥178

TABLE 2 (CONTINUED)

Desirable Weights for Women

Height Without Shoes	Frame Size	Desirable Weight (Pounds)	Overweight (≥20% over Desirable Weight)	Obese (≥30% over Desirable Weight)
5'5"	Small	118–127	≥146	≥159
5'5"	Medium	124–139	≥157	≥170
5'5"	Large	133–150	≥169	≥183
5'6"	Small	122–131	≥151	≥164
5'6"	Medium	128–143	≥162	≥176
5'6"	Large	137–154	≥174	≥188
5'7"	Small	126–135	≥156	≥169
5'7"	Medium	132–147	≥167	≥181
5'7"	Large	141–158	≥179	≥194
5'8"	Small	130–140	≥162	≥176
5'8"	Medium	136–151	≥172	≥186
5'8"	Large	145–163	≥185	≥200
5'9"	Small	134–144	≥167	≥181
5'9"	Medium	140–155	≥176	≥191
5'9"	Large	149–168	≥190	≥205
5'10"	Small	138–148	≥172	≥186
5'10"	Medium	144–159	≥181	≥196
5'10"	Large	153–173	≥196	≥212

Adapted from 1983 Metropolitan Life Insurance Company height/weight table, reprinted with permission, *Statistical Bulletin*, 1983.

Perhaps you are wondering why there is a range of healthy weights. This is explained by bone size. Just as some bridges are made with small or medium steel girders and some with larger ones, bones come in different sizes. And just as the size of a bridge's steel framework determines how much weight it can carry, bone size dictates how much weight a body can hold without difficulty. As you would imagine, people with bigger bones can accommodate weights at the higher end of the scale, while those with more delicate bone structure should aim for the weight on the lower end.

There are two ways to determine your bone size (if you want exact figures, use both methods to make sure you get the same answer):

1. The easy, measurement-free method: Place the thumb and index finger of one hand around your other wrist, where there is a bone on either side. Make sure your fingers don't slip off the bones, or you won't get a correct reading. If the thumb and index finger:

   - OVERLAP, you have a small frame;
   - JUST TOUCH, you have a medium frame;
   - FAIL TO MEET, you have a large frame.

2. The measurement technique: For this you need a flexible, non-stretch measuring tape, such as the type seamstresses use. Place the tape around the same place noted in method one and obtain a measurement. Use the numbers in Table 3 to determine your frame size. Note that wrist size generally varies with height, so be sure to find the row that corresponds to your height when matching your measurement to your frame size.

TABLE 3

Frame Size Based on Wrist Measurement

Height	Wrist Size in Inches That Indicates Small Frame	Wrist Size in Inches That Indicates Medium Frame	Wrist Size in Inches That Indicates Large Frame
Under 5'3"	Less than 5½	5½ to 5¾	Greater than 5¾
5'3" to 5'4"	Less than 6	6 to 6¼	Greater than 6¼
Over 5'4"	Less than 6¼	6¼ to 6½	Greater than 6½

What is the main difference between the weight tables of today and those of a decade ago? Basically, they aren't forgiving of the extra pounds of the passing years. At one time weight-loss experts thought it was okay for people to gain a few pounds with each extra decade of life. After all, our bodies naturally tend toward gaining weight as we age—for more than one reason. First of all, somewhere around the third or fourth decade of life, our bodies start losing muscle mass. That affects weight because muscle mass burns a certain amount of calories, and fat tissue burns infinitely fewer calories. While each pound of muscle burns 35 to 50 calories at rest, a pound of fat burns only 2 calories. In order to burn the maximum number of calories, it is important to have as much muscle tissue as possible. Unfortunately, Mother Nature doesn't make this very easy for us as she tries to convert muscle to fat while we age.

Another reason we tend to gain weight as we grow older is that the body's calorie-burning machinery becomes less efficient with age. Less able to handle large calorie bundles efficiently, the body takes the easy way out and simply turns them into fat. Putting extra calories into fat storage is bad news; as anyone who has ever put on extra pounds knows, it is so much easier to gain weight than it is to take it off.

Given that nearly everyone gains weight with age, we used to accommodate this in the weight tables by allowing a few extra pounds for people as they age. No longer are we lenient. Simply put, a weight limit is a weight limit, and violating it at any age means risking your health. Studies have demonstrated, for example, that a weight gain of even ten or fifteen pounds during or after middle age significantly increases the risk of developing diabetes and heart disease.

Body Mass Index. The many advances in studying and deciphering the effects of weight problems have given us a much greater understanding of this issue than when I first entered this field twenty-five years ago. One of the most powerful tools developed to assess the effect of weight on health is the body mass index, or BMI.

BMI, which is determined by an equation using height and weight, helps us understand how weight affects the body. It gives us a way to use the simple measures of height and weight to understand how excess fat impacts our health. Ideally, this impact is assessed by performing very complicated medical tests to determine how much of a person's weight is fat and how a person's body tolerates the weight they carry. The results of these tests help us determine a person's risk for disease and even death from diseases associated with weight. But these tests are very expensive, and they are rarely conducted except in research settings. Fortunately, though, we have performed enough of these tests during clinical studies to understand how weight affects health and have been able to translate the results of all these tests into BMI, which we have calculated for you in the following table.

New research tells us that the negative impact of obesity occurs at a lower BMI than we once thought. According to these data we know that the risks of heart disease and diabetes begin to rise dramatically when BMI exceeds 25. Xenical is recommended when BMI equals or exceeds either 27 or 30.

- 27 applies when an overweight person has high blood pressure, high blood cholesterol, and/or diabetes. At this point we say the health risk of increased body weight, in combination with these other conditions, is great enough to warrant the use of Xenical.

- 30 applies when a person falls into the obese range but does not necessarily have other conditions such as high blood pressure, high blood cholesterol, or diabetes. Although these other conditions may not yet have occurred, a person this much over their healthy weight range is at high risk of developing other health problems, and use of Xenical is warranted to bring weight down before such conditions strike.

Waist Circumference. Ever heard the terms "apple" and "pear" used to describe a person's torso? These terms are not only graphically descriptive but also describe disease risk. Where a person's fat is stored is just as important as how much fat he or she carries. Specifically, we know that people with a lot of fat in their midsections (the apples of the world, who are more frequently men) are far more likely to suffer high blood pressure and heart disease than pear-shaped people (usually women) whose fat is on their hips and thighs. "Apples" also have more trouble with high triglyceride levels, a condition similar to having high cholesterol levels. Worse yet, these problems can accelerate quite dramatically even in relatively normal weight people if they are unfortunate enough to carry excess fat around their middles. The number we use to assess the risk of midsection fatness is called the waist circumference.

(We used to use another figure to assess a person's abdominal fat—the waist-to-hip ratio, or WHR—but waist circumference has been found to be a better marker of abdominal fat content.)

It is easy to determine your own waist circumference. Simply measure around the widest point between the top of your hips and the bottom of your rib cage. Draw the tape snugly but not tight; it should not compress the skin. Measure during a normal breath.

The ideal waist circumference varies by gender. To reduce the chance of developing risk factors for heart disease and diabetes, men should strive for a waist circumference of less than 40 inches, and women should strive for a waist circumference of less than 35 inches.

Comorbid Conditions. This term refers to the presence of risk factors for disease or the diseases themselves, including those already mentioned here and earlier in the book: high blood cholesterol, high blood pressure, and diabetes. Xenical is recommended at a lower BMI when a person has at least one of these comorbid conditions because we know that weight has adversely affected health when weight-related diseases have already struck.

How to Determine BMI

This chart will help you determine your BMI (body mass index), which indicates the relationship between your weight and your height. Find your height on the side, locate your weight in the top row, and move down and across until the columns meet. The resulting number, at the intersection, is your BMI measurement.

A BMI equal to or greater than 25 means that you are overweight and have a greater risk of developing some of the conditions associated with obesity such as high blood pressure, heart disease, and adult-onset (type 2) diabetes. Obesity is defined as the point at which a person's BMI is equal to or greater than 30.

Weight (pounds)

	120	130	140	150	160	170	180	190	200	210	220	230	240	250	260	270	280	290	300	310	320	330
4'5"	30	33	35	38	40	43	45	48	50	53	55	58	60	63	65	68	70	73	75	78	80	83
4'6"	29	31	34	36	39	41	43	46	48	51	53	56	58	60	63	65	68	70	72	75	77	80
4'7"	28	30	33	35	37	40	42	44	47	49	51	54	56	58	61	63	65	68	70	72	75	77
4'8"	27	29	31	34	36	38	40	43	45	47	49	52	54	56	58	61	63	65	67	70	72	74
4'9"	26	28	30	33	35	37	39	41	43	46	48	50	52	54	56	59	61	63	65	67	69	72
4'10"	25	27	29	31	34	36	38	40	42	44	46	48	50	52	54	57	59	61	63	65	67	69
4'11"	24	26	28	30	32	34	36	38	40	43	45	47	49	51	53	55	57	59	61	63	65	67
5'0"	23	25	27	29	31	33	35	37	39	41	43	45	47	49	51	53	55	57	59	61	63	65
5'1"	23	25	27	28	30	32	34	36	38	40	42	44	45	47	49	51	53	55	57	59	61	62
5'2"	22	24	26	27	29	31	33	35	37	38	40	42	44	46	48	49	51	53	55	57	59	60
5'3"	21	23	25	27	28	30	32	34	36	37	39	41	43	44	46	48	50	51	53	55	57	59
5'4"	21	22	24	26	28	29	31	33	34	36	38	40	41	43	45	46	48	50	52	53	55	57

Height																						
5'5"	20	22	23	25	27	28	30	32	33	35	37	38	40	42	43	45	47	48	50	52	53	55
5'6"	19	21	23	24	26	27	29	31	32	34	36	37	39	40	42	44	45	47	49	50	52	53
5'7"	19	20	22	24	25	27	28	30	31	33	35	36	38	39	41	42	44	46	47	49	50	52
5'8"	18	20	21	23	24	26	27	29	30	32	34	35	37	38	40	41	43	44	46	47	49	50
5'9"	18	19	21	22	24	25	27	28	30	31	33	34	36	37	38	40	41	43	44	46	47	49
5'10"	17	19	20	22	23	24	26	27	29	30	32	33	35	36	37	39	40	42	43	45	46	47
5'11"	17	18	20	21	22	23	25	26	28	29	31	32	34	35	36	38	39	41	42	43	45	46
6'0"	16	18	19	20	21	22	24	25	27	29	30	31	33	34	35	37	38	39	41	42	43	45
6'1"	16	17	19	20	21	22	24	24	26	28	29	30	32	33	34	36	37	38	40	41	42	44
6'2"	15	17	18	19	20	21	23	24	25	27	28	29	31	32	33	35	36	37	39	40	41	42
6'3"	15	16	18	19	20	21	23	23	24	26	28	28	30	31	33	34	35	36	38	39	40	41
6'4"	15	16	17	18	19	20	22	22	24	26	27	28	30	30	32	33	34	35	37	38	39	40
6'5"	14	15	17	18	19	20	21	22	23	25	26	27	29	30	31	32	33	34	36	37	38	39
6'6"	14	15	16	17	19	20	21	21	23	24	25	26	28	29	30	31	32	34	35	36	37	38
6'7"	14	15	16	17	18	19	20	21	22	24	25	26	27	28	30	31	32	33	34	35	36	37
6'8"	13	14	15	17	18	19	20	20	22	23	24	25	26	28	29	30	31	32	33	34	35	36
6'9"	13	14	15	16	17	18	19	20	21	23	24	24	26	27	28	29	30	31	32	33	34	35
6'10"	13	14	15	16	17	18	19	20	21	22	23	23	25	26	27	28	29	30	31	32	34	35

Is Xenical Right for Me?

Answer the questions on this worksheet to help you decide whether Xenical is right for you.

1. In what category does your body weight place you?
   Normal weight_____
   Overweight_____
   Obese_____

If you answered overweight or obese, you may be a candidate for Xenical. Go on to Question 2.

2. Do you have high blood pressure, high blood cholesterol, and/or diabetes?
   Yes_____
   No_____

3. If you answered yes, is your BMI 27 or greater?
   Yes_____
   No_____

If you have at least one of these comorbid conditions and your BMI is 27 or greater, you may be a candidate for Xenical.

4. If you answered no, is your BMI 30 or greater?
   Yes_____
   No_____

If you do not have a comorbid condition but your BMI is 30 or greater, you are at high risk of health problems from your weight and may be a candidate for Xenical.

5. What is your waist circumference?

Men:

a. Under 40 inches_____

b. 40 inches or above_____

Women:

a. Under 35 inches_____

b. 35 inches or above_____

If you selected category b, your risk of disease is particularly great if you also determined that you are in the obese range in question 1 and/or that you are at high risk for complications from your weight in question 2.

Issues to Discuss with Your Doctor

Discuss with the physician who prescribes Xenical for you all medical conditions you have now or have ever had as well as every medication you take. This is especially important if the doctor you see for weight loss is different from your regular family doctor and therefore doesn't know your medical history. If you are planning to adopt a new exercise routine, such as one of those described in chapter 6, be sure to let your doctor know.

It is important that you not take Xenical if you

- have a chronic malabsorption condition, meaning that your gastrointestinal tract does not absorb nutrients as well as it should; for example if you have Crohn's disease or if you have had some of your bowel surgically removed;
- have cholestasis (blocked bile ducts);
- have had an allergic reaction to Xenical;
- are pregnant or nursing. Also, since Xenical has not yet been tested in people under eighteen or over sixty-five, recommendations cannot be made for people in these age groups.

The Principles of the Xenical Program

If, in conjunction with your doctor, you've decided to take Xenical to aid your weight-loss efforts, make a commitment that is even greater: commit yourself not just to the Xenical pill but to the Xenical program. Cindy, the patient you met in the introduction, lost only part of her weight—forty-seven of the total seventy pounds—while taking Xenical. "I learned that to lose weight I had to transform my total way of life. Xenical gave me the confidence to do that," says Cindy, who has maintained a healthful and trim weight for three years. She has not taken Xenical for four years.

As Cindy learned, several principles of the Xenical program are keys to success:

- Take the correct dose of Xenical at the correct times.
- Eat healthy foods with an appropriate fat content at each meal.
- Eat low-fat snacks between meals.

- Take the recommended vitamin and mineral supplements.
- Design an exercise program you can stick with over the long haul.
- Learn to like yourself today, at your current weight, rather than waiting until you achieve a certain weight.

Taking Xenical Properly

Because taking Xenical properly is so important to success, I would like to spend some time discussing how to do this.

As you fill your first prescription for Xenical and then open the bottle for the first time, print indelibly on your brain one very important fact: Xenical is a drug. Just as you make every effort to take other prescription medications properly so that they can have the desired effect without problems, do the same with Xenical. It is human nature to regard weight-loss aids, even prescription medications, with less seriousness than medication to control high blood pressure, for example, but misusing a weight-loss aid such as Xenical may also have serious consequences.

These are the four things you need to do to take Xenical properly:

1. Take only the prescribed dose. Your physician will probably prescribe 120-milligram tablets to be taken three times daily.

2. Take the tablets at the correct time. With some medications it doesn't matter if you take them on an empty or a full stomach. Not so with Xenical. Since the drug is designed to stop some of the fat in your meals from being absorbed, it has to be in the intestinal tract when you eat fat-containing meals. The best time to take Xenical is at the beginning of a meal so that it can go to work immediately to inhibit fat absorption. If you are planning to dine out, don't take the pill before leaving the house because too much time may pass before you get your meal, and Xenical may lose its effectiveness before your food is served. Like any pill, Xenical has a limited "therapeutic window," meaning that it works for only a short time once inside the body.

3. Follow the diet properly. Limit yourself to the prescribed amount of fat. Some people think that because Xenical inhibits fat absorption, they can eat all the fat they want and suffer no consequences, but they find that Xenical may work to corral the fat calories for a price. There is only one place for Xenical to dump the excess

fat, and that is in the intestinal tract. The result of eating too much fat can be intestinal discomfort. This might include the need to have a bowel movement quickly and loose, oily stools. Some people may notice bloating and oily spotting.

4. Take a vitamin/mineral supplement that supplies 100 percent of the U.S. Recommended Dietary Allowance (RDA) for all essential nutrients. The reason is that Xenical decreases fat absorption, so it may decrease the absorption of fat-soluble vitamins. Don't take more than the RDA because your body will excrete the excess. Take your vitamin/mineral supplement with one of your snacks for maximum absorption. Since it doesn't matter which snack, just choose one for consistency. Otherwise take the supplement at bedtime. Fat-soluble vitamins are so named because they piggyback onto dietary fat to be absorbed. Extensive research has shown that taking a vitamin/mineral supplement that supplies 100 percent of the U.S. RDA for all nutrients is more than sufficient to make up for any possible losses that occur with Xenical (refer to chapter 3 for details). As a weight-loss expert who has analyzed dieters' eating behaviors for over a quarter-century, I also know that people fully committed to eating better, not just losing weight, give themselves a nutrient advantage. Because they adopt a much healthier diet overall, they almost always take in more vitamins and minerals. This, too, helps offset the losses experienced while taking Xenical.

The Xenical Diet and Exercise Program: An Overview

Chapters 3, 4, and 5 describe how to eat while taking Xenical for maximum benefit, and chapter 6 outlines the exercise program that best complements your efforts. Briefly, this is what you need to do:

- Eat the prescribed amount of dietary fat (no more than 30 percent of a day's total calories) at the appropriate times throughout the day. It is not enough just to limit total fat grams for the day, though. It matters when you eat fat and how much you eat at any one time. Chapter 4 shows you exactly how to eat this way and gives many menu ideas and exciting new recipes that will make following this healthy dietary program possible for as long as necessary.
- Do not skimp on calories. We know from experience that it is not necessary to eliminate calories so drastically that you become so

hungry that you binge. We recommend eliminating about 600 calories from your current day's total and show you how to calculate
this in chapter 3.

- Eat very low-fat snacks. You'll be taking Xenical only with meals
so it will only block fat absorption from those meals. As mentioned
earlier, Xenical doesn't work long enough to stop fat absorption
from the snacks you eat between meals.

- Track what you eat. To achieve success at challenging ventures, it
is important to use every tool available to you. Tracking what you
eat by using a food diary is a tremendous help in losing weight
steadily and consistently. A food diary is provided in chapter 5.

- Exercise regularly. The human body naturally wants to conserve
energy, which means that every time we eat less than our body
requires to maintain weight—in other words, any time we diet—
the body wants to turn down its metabolic rate (the rate at which
it burns calories). But exercising alters this survival strategy and
turns the metabolic rate back up. There are several other reasons
to exercise regularly, and these will be discussed in chapter 6.

Using Xenical with Other Diets

There is tremendous merit in many other weight-loss programs available on the market. Some of these programs, such as Weight Watchers
and Jenny Craig, offer emotional support, camaraderie, and dietary
instruction to help you achieve success. It is not necessary for you to
enroll in one of their programs if you decide to try Xenical, but it is certainly all right to do so if you think it might be helpful. Another possibility is to enlist the help of a registered dietitian (RD). An RD is the
ultimately knowledgeable healthcare professional when it comes to
food, eating, and the effect of nutrition on good health. He or she can
help you translate nutrition information into real-life eating practices.

If you use any of these other weight-loss programs, you may have to
modify them slightly so that Xenical has the maximum benefit—and to
reduce the risk of suffering side effects. These other programs often
allow a certain amount of fat for the whole day and let you eat it whenever you choose. If you wanted to save your fat grams for a bowl of ice
cream and hot fudge sauce, for example, you could do that on these
plans. Not so with Xenical. Saving all your fat grams for one indulgence
during the day could have unpleasant consequences, resulting in intestinal discomfort and other gastrointestinal problems as described in the
previous chapter.

In general, to modify these other programs, you'll have to:

1. Make sure fat calories don't exceed 30 percent of a day's total calorie intake and then divide them evenly among three meals. As with the Xenical diet and exercise plan, don't exceed an absolute number of 20 fat grams at any one meal;

2. Choose snack foods that are very low in fat or fat free;

3. Be wary of any diet plan that is extremely low in calories, as some programs are. We do not recommend dropping below 1,200 calories per day and feel strongly that you will have greater success at around 1,500 calories.

Let's take a look at some specific programs and how to use them with Xenical.

Xenical with Weight Watchers

The Weight Watchers program changes from time to time, so you'll have to determine how to count fat grams at each meal and in snacks if you're going to combine Weight Watchers with Xenical. The Weight Watchers program may have distinct rules for how you can use the foods allowed; for example, you may be able to divide up your food throughout the day however you desire. But this won't work if you are taking Xenical.

First, figure out which foods in their program have fat grams (they typically divide food up by categories). Distribute the fat-containing foods in the diet plan evenly throughout breakfast, lunch, and dinner. Do not exceed 20 grams of fat at any one meal. If there is more fat in the diet plan, you'll have to substitute lower-fat foods for some of these foods so that you don't exceed 20 fat grams.

For snack foods use only those foods on the plan that have few or negligible fat grams. You may want to save some of your fruit servings and nonfat dairy foods for snacks. Incidentally, be sure to have snack foods while on the Xenical plan. Even though other plans, such as Weight Watchers, do not always require you to eat foods in between meals, we know from experience that you may have greater success in losing weight if you eat smaller meals and save some of your calories for snacks.

Xenical with Jenny Craig

In dieting with Jenny Craig, you typically purchase some prepared foods in specific serving sizes (the great value is that you stick to one portion size and become accustomed to the concept of portion sizes). Along with these prepared foods you often add your own fruits, salads, and fat-free dairy foods. To use the Jenny Craig system with Xenical, simply tally the number of fat grams you are using at each meal and do not exceed 20 grams per meal. The foods you add—fruit, vegetables, and fat-free dairy—contain few, if any, fat grams, so you don't have to tally them.

As for snack foods, use only the low-fat foods we've been recommending—fruit, vegetables, and fat-free dairy. If there are dessert foods on the program with fat grams, use them with your meals and tally them as part of the 20-gram total.

Xenical with the National Cholesterol Education Program (NCEP)

If you have high cholesterol levels, your doctor may recommend that you follow either the Step I or Step II NCEP diet. Fortunately, both of these work well if you decide to take Xenical. They have 30 percent of calories from fat for the day, at most. The only thing you may have to modify is how you divide up your fat. This program doesn't necessarily divide up fat evenly throughout your meals, which you will have to do with Xenical. Also, this eating plan allows snacks with higher amounts of fat grams, which are not recommended if you are taking Xenical. Just move all of these foods into your three meals, making sure that no one meal exceeds 20 grams of fat, and concentrate on very low fat foods for snacks between meals.

Although the rules for using Xenical optimally and safely are very specific, they are few in number. We hope you will find them easy now that we've explained them thoroughly. As with any drug, we know you can make Xenical work for you as long as you take it properly and follow the food instructions. With this background, let's move on to the specifics of dieting and exercising when on Xenical.

3

Dieting with Xenical: The Principles

It's a typical work day for forty-four-year-old Margaret: hurry to get the kids off to school with little time for a decent breakfast, no time to pack a lunch for work, and just enough time after work for a "thirty-minute dinner." Despite her harried life, there is something fabulously positive about Margaret. She's making an incredible effort to adopt a new eating style, one with healthier foods and fewer calories so that she can lose the forty pounds that crept on over the past fifteen years. Most of all, she is trying to make the smart changes that will take her off the lose-gain treadmill that has all but sapped her last bit of dieting energy.

Wanting to lose weight quickly in the past, Margaret went on so-called crash diets, or eating plans that supply a measly 1,000 calories. After so many years of this starvation torture, she knows the consequences: bingeing. Margaret has found that going below 1,500 calories daily backfires on her efforts—and in a big hurry. By late afternoon or evening of the first or second day of skimping on food, Margaret is so ravenous that she satisfies her pangs with ice cream or chips, and frequently blows her entire day's success in fifteen minutes of reckless eating abandon.

Even when Margaret can stay with 1,200 or so calories for a week or two and enjoys a more rapid weight loss—about three or four pounds a week for a while—her body outsmarts her. Like any body starved for food (and it doesn't distinguish between when it is starved for food because of famine and when it is starved by design to become thin), Margaret's undernourished body powers down to its conservation mode. The human body has an amazing ability to sense that calories are scarce, so it turns down its metabolism to save precious energy in the hope of getting through the calorie deficit without losing body mass. This worked for our ancient ancestors who couldn't afford to lose weight and didn't have a supermarket or McDonald's just down the road, but this hangover survival strategy makes weight loss very difficult today and defeats the efforts of the disciplined dieter.

Over Margaret's long and frustrating dieting career, she has come to realize that settling on a 1,500-calorie weight-loss diet is in her best interest. It saves her from rebound eating out of pure hunger and prevents her body from powering down into starvation conservation. But Margaret discovered another critically essential need, one she cannot ignore at any point of her life but most especially when she is dieting. She needs to stop engaging in a battle with food, to cease thinking of it as the enemy. This discovery also keeps Margaret from bingeing. Thankfully, Margaret now approaches food as humans are meant to: she enjoys the food she eats—every single bite.

Food and the Head

Margaret has come to the realization that eating is meant to satisfy more than pure physical and nutritional needs. Food also assuages psychological and human needs. We don't often think about food as the pleasurable entity it was meant to be, especially if we are constantly engaged in a battle with food as the enemy. This occurs so often to dieters because food is a major struggle in their lives. But it is possible to get over this hurdle; it is possible to eat enough food to feel satisfied and content and yet lose weight.

The key word is balance, not just in nutrients but in emotional satisfaction. When you find the right balance, you'll revel in an exceptionally pleasant feeling that most dieters no longer experience. Because Margaret and other dieters have become strangers to the enjoyment of food, they have left themselves vulnerable to another form of bingeing: filling in the pleasure gaps left by eating food that does not satisfy the multiple senses, which are such an important part of eating.

In our society, food was never meant to have just one purpose; it was never intended just to feed and energize the body. Instead, our culture has given it an exceptionally complex set of values: food celebrates life and success, it heals physical wounds and emotional trauma, and it marks anniversaries and death. Thus, the birth of such terms as "comfort foods"—the foods people turn to in times of emotional turmoil, with ice cream, chocolate, and macaroni and cheese at the top of the list.

This is why it is so important to acknowledge the other purposes of food and make certain you eat the food you love.

Margaret has come to accept that she can lose weight on a diet that doesn't leave her starving, ready to binge, or emotionally deprived. A bonus of this acceptance is that Margaret not only can lose steadily but can lose a little faster with Xenical. Let's look at what makes up the food we eat and then discuss dieting.

Food Is More than Calories: Understanding Food

Many Americans have gotten confused about food. In years gone by we ate for sustenance and enjoyment, and then there was a gradual transition to the "good food/bad food" concept. Unfortunately, we've come to think that good food is synonymous with high-calorie, decadent choices not compatible with healthy living. On the other hand, "being good" means that you are eating celery sticks, rice cakes, and broiled chicken breasts that have taken on the consistency of dry hockey pucks.

The good news is that nutrition professionals are bridging the gap between what is good for you and what delights the taste buds. And that brings a whole new dimension to dieting.

Before explaining the fascinating world of food and why your body needs it, let me help you jump over the "good food/bad food" hurdle. You'll then be in a world where food is good for you and delights the taste buds with every bite. This is the beginning of not feeling deprived when you make the transition to eating in a slimmer way.

Close your eyes and imagine a perfect autumn day. With your mind's paintbrush, splash together every shade of yellow, red, orange, purple, brown, and the thousands of shades of green that only Mother Nature can create, each color bursting into the next to create the ultimate still-life portrait. Now imagine the almost magical and certainly complex process orchestrated by Mother Nature to produce that scene. Close your eyes again and turn that still-life portrait into a fiesta of nature's gastronomical treasures: sweet papaya, succulent tomatoes, robust whole wheat bread with a swirl of rich peanut butter, honey-flavored tangerines, dulcet grapes, peppery but soft watercress, nutty brown rice with cilantro sauce. Does this food make you feel deprived? I hope not! Now, let's move on to a quick nutrition lesson about carbohydrates, protein, and fat.

Three Kinds of Calories. The body uses three kinds of calories, called macronutrients: carbohydrates, protein, and fat. Each is different from the others, and one cannot replace another. That is why it is so important not to regard fat calories as the ultimate enemy or as the only type of calorie to be controlled.

Gaining Weight the Fat-Free Way

As Americans have become more and more confused about food, many people have come to regard fat calories as the only calories that need to be controlled. Thus, we have come to demand fat-free foods. Industry has responded to this clamoring demand by creating a great variety of fat-free foods. Americans now eat plenty of these foods—including fat-free pretzels, coffee cakes, and cookies—but the trouble is that we are not losing weight on these fat-free foods. In fact, Americans are continuing to gain weight, partly because people sometimes forget that fat-free foods can still be high in calories. That is why it is important for you to understand that the human body will gain weight on any type of calorie you eat in excess. You need to understand how to eat for good health, not just count fat grams. This is part of making Xenical work to your best advantage.

Carbohydrates. Carbohydrates are the premium form of energy, or fuel, for the human body. You may know carbohydrates by other names, such as starch, sugar, and glucose. Sugar is a confusing term; Americans use it to refer to many things, but it is just the common word used for "carbohydrates." Starch and glucose are two terms that describe different forms of carbohydrates (which come from "carbo," for the carbon it contains, and "hydrate," for its hydrogen atoms). Each gram of carbohydrate has about 4 calories.

Glucose is one of the simplest sugars found in food, having just a single molecule. It is the form of sugar to which all other types of sugar are eventually converted in the body. Think of glucose as one link in a chain fence. It is also the form of sugar carried in the bloodstream as the ultimate energy source that jumpstarts cells, keeps us thinking clearly, and fuels our muscles. Fructose and galactose are other simple sugars found in foods such as fruit. All simple, one-molecule sugars are called monosaccharides ("mono" meaning one and "saccharide" meaning sugar).

Next on the carbohydrate ladder are the disaccharides ("di" stands for two). As you imagine disaccharides, think of two links on a chain fence joined together. Disaccharides are two simple sugars hooked together. Sucrose, the chemical name for table sugar, is one example of a disaccharide.

At the top of the heap are the polysaccharides, or substances with many simple sugars joined together. An image of polysaccharides would be tens or even hundreds of the links in a chain fence joined together. Rice, wheat, potatoes, and soybeans are just some of the many foods containing polysaccharides, which are also called starch.

But how do the terms "simple" and "complex" carbohydrates come into play? Complex carbohydrate foods are made up primarily of poly-saccharides. These foods are complex in terms of how they are formed and also because wrapped into their elaborate packages are lots of vit-amins, minerals, sometimes protein (such as the complex carbohydrate foods lentils and split peas), and fiber, plus many health benefits. When we eat starchy foods, we benefit from the entire nutritional package, not just the polysaccharides.

Simple carbohydrates are foods containing monosaccharides or di-saccharides. Very sweet in flavor, they include such favorite treats as honey, syrup, candy, desserts, soda pop, and sweetened cereals. We know that complex carbohydrates are by far the best choice, but are sugary foods or simple carbohydrates bad for your health, as you may have read? Only in the sense that they may keep you from eating better foods and fill you up quite quickly on "empty" calories. Most simple carbohydrate foods have very few, if any, nutrients other than calories because the sugars are refined, or unwrapped from that com-plex carbohydrate package. Put another way, sugar is stripped from its source, leaving behind the vitamins, minerals, and fiber and taking only the calories.

Carbohydrates should make up the bulk of your daily eating plan. Approximately 50 to 60 percent of your daily calories should come from car-bohydrates. At least four of five carbohydrate calories (or 80 percent) should be complex. Currently, Americans eat about half of their carbohydrates as the simple carbohydrates table sugar and high-fructose corn syrup, which are used to sweeten such items as soda pop, cereals, fruit juices, and yogurts. That means Americans eat the equivalent of more than sixteen teaspoons of sugar each day, or sixty pounds of table sugar and fifty pounds of corn syrup each year. In contrast, one hundred years ago, the average American consumed just four pounds of table sugar in an entire year. What I find fascinating is that many people in developing countries actually eat healthier than we do: their dietary staples of rice and beans take them much closer to healthier eating.

The eating plans we have designed for you in chapter 4 include just the right amounts of the complex carbohydrates you need for good health. As a general guideline, though, to help you choose foods yourself, here is how to plan your own complex carbohydrate intake:

- Cereal grains: included among the common varieties are wheat, rye, rice, corn, and oats. Among the not so common are barley, quinoa, and millet. Try them as the whole grain, either as a side dish or in a casserole, or try breads and bagels made from their flours. Depending on your calorie level, you'll have five to ten servings of grain foods each day in which one serving is ½ cup of cooked grain or 1 ounce of a bagel/bread product.
- Legumes: sample all the nutrient-packed carbs—black beans, chickpeas, kidney beans, brown and red lentils, soybeans (as the bean or tofu), and peanuts. You should have at least one serving daily of ½ cup of cooked legume.
- Vegetables: have at least five servings of several different types of vegetables daily, such as green leafy (romaine lettuce, spinach), yellow/red (carrots, winter squash), and cruciferous (broccoli, cauliflower, Brussels sprouts). You should divide the vegetables into starchy ones (which count toward your grain food servings) and those much lower in calories. Here are some general guidelines:
  - Starchy vegetables: peas, corns, potatoes, sweet potatoes, lima beans.
  - Lower-calorie vegetables: includes everything green, leafy, or stalky, such as lettuce, broccoli, cauliflower, onions, leeks, and asparagus.
- Fruits: try every kind of fruit, aiming for three to five servings daily, depending on your calorie level. Choose any fruit, including berries, melons, apples, citrus, cherries, and peaches. Although you may think of fruits as simple sugars, they come wrapped in a valuable nutritional package full of vitamins, minerals, fiber, and those hot new nutritional substances called phytochemicals that confer many health benefits.

Later you will learn how to choose carbohydrate foods without getting the excess fat that often accompanies them.

Protein. Protein is confusing today, especially with the reemergence of the high-protein diet. Before we look at the dangers of high-protein diets, let's review some protein basics.

Like carbohydrates, proteins contain approximately 4 calories per gram. Protein is constructed of building blocks called amino acids. Like carbohydrates and fats, amino acids are made of carbon, hydrogen, and oxygen molecules, but an additional element, nitrogen, distinguishes protein from these other energy sources. The amino acids are joined together in thousands of ways to form long chains called peptides. Two proteins may have totally different functions—liver protein and muscle protein, for example—but be composed of exactly the same amino acids. The difference lies in how these amino acids are linked together.

There are two categories of amino acids: essential and nonessential. These categories have nothing to do with how important each is in the human body; rather, the categories distinguish between those amino acids the body can make and those it cannot. Of the twenty-two amino acids needed by the human body, nine are dietary essentials, meaning they must come from the food we eat. The remaining thirteen are nonessential dietary components because the body can make them from scraps of leftover carbohydrates, fats, and other amino acids.

If you lack just one essential amino acid for any period of time, no matter what quantity of other amino acids you eat, your body will break down its own protein tissue to harvest that essential amino acid so it can build hormones and perform functions more vital than building and maintaining muscle tissue. If this process continues, you may suffer the effects of protein malnutrition, which, in addition to loss of muscle mass, include thin, fragile hair (or hair loss); skin sores; swelling; and one of many chemical and hormonal imbalances. Fortunately, protein deficiency of this severity is rare, especially in the United States.

Protein-containing foods can be divided into two main categories, complete proteins and incomplete proteins, based on what kinds of amino acids they contain or their amino acid mix. Foods containing all essential amino acids are called complete proteins; these are generally animal proteins such as meat, chicken, fish, milk, cheese, and eggs. If one or more essential amino acids are lacking, that protein is termed incomplete. Most protein from animal sources is complete, and most protein from plant sources is incomplete. Other foods, such as soybeans and many nuts, can be said to be "weakly complete"; that is, they contain all essential amino acids but don't have enough of one or more to assemble body proteins. Fortunately, though, these incomplete or weakly complete protein foods can be used as complete protein sources.

With a little dietary maneuvering, one incomplete protein food can be combined with another incomplete protein food to make up for the other's deficiency. This is called "complementing proteins." The trick is to make correct combinations. Until recently, nutrition experts thought incomplete proteins had to be complemented within the same meal to ensure their use as protein rather than just calories. More recent research reveals, however, that incomplete protein foods only need to be complemented within twenty-four hours. Eating a very small quantity of a complete protein food with an incomplete one—a glass of milk (complete protein) with a bowl of lentil soup (incomplete protein), for example—also ensures that the protein in the incomplete protein food is converted to a high-quality protein. Here are some other ways to complement proteins:

- corn tortilla and pinto beans
- peanut butter on whole wheat bread
- bulgur wheat and red lentils
- navy bean soup and rye bread

As was said earlier, the danger lies in eating too much protein, especially with the emergence of high-protein diets. My opinion is that these diets, which emerged in the seventies, weren't good then and aren't beneficial now. High-protein/low-carbohydrate diets have come and gone over the past quarter-century. They are based on the belief that many people suffer a carbohydrate allergy, or at least a "sugar imbalance," if they eat carbohydrates. Either condition makes weight loss difficult, say the proponents.

Such diets permit people to eat all the protein and fatty foods they want, including beef, pork, chicken, bacon, butter, sour cream, and cheese, while they prohibit corn, bananas, apples, rice, pasta, and whole grains. Proponents believe that substituting protein for carbohydrate calories should reduce the body's production of insulin, which increases appetite and fat storage. However, protein stimulates insulin production, especially in the context of a mixed meal (one that contains carbohydrates, protein, and fat). Preliminary evidence suggests that on a gram-for-gram basis, protein may stimulate more insulin than carbohydrate. Overall, high-protein diets are nutritionally dangerous—especially for people with heart disease. This is because the fat content tends to be high; they are also quite low in the nutrient-rich carbohydrate foods that are so important to good health. The high-protein content is certainly not good for people with compromised kidney function because all the excess protein in these diets must be filtered out through the kidneys. One last word: the American Heart Association, the American Diabetes Association, and other official groups advise against such diets.

The most important advice about protein is to get the amount you need without excess fat. The best way to do this is to eat a wide variety of protein foods and limit portion sizes. I am certain that many Americans unconsciously overeat foods rich in protein. Rethink protein-rich foods as the garnish to your meal rather than the focus. You'll automatically cut calories. Aim for three ounces of chicken at a main meal, rather than the four- to six-ounce portion that most people eat.

Some other goals for eating protein foods wisely are as follows:

- Try to have no more than one or two red meat dinners weekly (beef, pork, or veal), two to four ounces in each serving. Also try to limit skinless poultry meals to two weekly, two to four ounces in each serving. Get the rest of your protein foods from fish or vegetable sources.
- Make an effort to substitute meatless meals for those containing meat. This will greatly reduce your fat intake (particularly those heart unhealthy fats, saturated fat and cholesterol). Non-meat sources of protein, including legumes and nuts, also provide heart-disease-fighting substances, such as fiber, vitamins, and minerals. Remember, when you eat well and feel better, you eat less; that is, your battery is better charged.
- Prepare some fish meals. Fish provides omega-3 fatty acids. This type of fat, which is unique to fish, flaxseed, and a few dark green leafy vegetables, helps prevent heart disease by keeping platelets from clumping together too much; it also raises HDL, or good cholesterol. Other evidence suggests that it may reduce inflammatory processes, such as those involved in arthritis. More fish also means less saturated and total fat in the diet. Aim to eat at least two fish meals weekly, three to five ounces in each serving.
- For lunch, try to choose vegetable sources of protein, such as garbanzo beans, black beans, soy nuts, peanut butter, and split peas.

Fat. As was said previously, fat calories are necessary. It is important to limit them, especially while taking Xenical, but some fat is necessary to good health. Without fat, the body's billions of cells could neither form properly nor regulate the entry and exit of nutrients, hormones, and other life-essential chemicals. Vital internal organs might suffer serious injury in its absence. Hormones couldn't form or function, nor could the body harness, transport, and use certain vitamins without fat.

In the fervor to reduce dietary fat, Americans are forgetting a crucial fact: it's the dose that makes the poison. Consider this analogy: aspirin can lower a fever and relieve pain at the right dose, but it's harmful at higher doses. The same is true of many nutrients and chemicals. Too much salt and even too much water can be fatal. But, like fat, they are crucial to the human body.

On the other hand, fat is the most calorically dense food substance we eat, supplying about 9 calories per gram. That's 2.25 times the calories we get from carbohydrates and protein (and that's why a little piece of fat-rich chocolate can do so much damage), yet the overconsumption of fat is the most important dietary mistake made in this country. As a nation we eat some 839 billion fat calories each year.

Chemically speaking, fat is just one substance within a larger category of substances called lipids. Oily or greasy to the touch and insoluble in water, lipids include dietary fats such as cooking oil, butter, lard, and the fat that is an inherent part of many meats, dairy products, and other foods. Also included in this lipid category are hormones, waxes, and sterols. Cholesterol is the best known sterol. Not a dietary fat at all, it's a fatlike substance present in all animal cells. Cholesterol does not supply calories because it is not composed of the same energy-supplying compounds as fats and oils. Surprisingly, the majority of the cholesterol in our bodies is formed within the body itself, with saturated fat as the primary building block.

Fat is formed from the same basic ingredients found in nature as are protein and carbohydrates: carbon, hydrogen, and oxygen. The difference is in the proportions and how the basic ingredients are connected. Fats contain much less oxygen than do proteins and carbohydrates. Simply put, the air is squeezed out of fat, which makes it a more compact source of energy.

Dietary fats consist mainly of units called triglycerides, which are made up of one glycerol molecule connected to three fatty acids. The most important structural feature of a triglyceride is the fatty acid portion. This is the segment that distinguishes one type of triglyceride, or dietary fat, from another, both in terms of flavor and the fat's effect within the human body. Some fatty acids are saturated, some are monounsaturated, and others are polyunsaturated. Saturation simply refers to how much hydrogen a fat contains. Saturated fatty acids are saturated with hydrogen, or contain the maximum amount of hydrogen atoms possible. Fats missing one pair of hydrogen atoms are monounsaturated; those missing more than one pair are polyunsaturated. Although they differ by just a couple of hydrogen atoms, these different types of fat behave quite differently in the body.

Any food that contains fat has all three types of fatty acids, but generally one type predominates. Dietary fats are generally called by the name of the predominating fat. Olive oil, for example, is deemed a "monounsaturated" fat because 75 percent of its fatty acids are monounsaturated. However, it also contains some polyunsaturated and a little saturated fat. Fats that contain predominantly polyunsaturated and monounsaturated fatty acids are liquid at room temperature. Saturated fats are solid. Picture a bottle of liquid olive oil versus the white waxy layer of saturated fat on a platter of cooling roast beef. As a rule, fats of plant origin, such as vegetable oils, are almost entirely poly and mono (the only two exceptions are coconut and palm oils, which are predominantly saturated fat). Animal fats—those in dairy foods, beef, pork, and chicken—are predominantly saturated.

This clear animal/plant demarcation is highly significant when it comes to choosing a better fat. Vegetable fats are always better than animal fats. Or, in terms of the type of fat, monos and polys are much better choices than saturated fats.

Saturated fat is the heart's greatest food enemy. It is the most significant dietary culprit in raising blood cholesterol levels, especially LDL cholesterol, the cholesterol that builds up on arterial walls and narrows them. One of the ways saturated fat is thought to raise LDL cholesterol levels is by impairing the liver's cholesterol removal machinery. Normally, LDL receptors stand ready like large grappling hooks on the end of liver cells, ready to snag LDL cholesterol as it flows by; the LDL particles are then packaged for removal from the body via the intestinal tract. Saturated fat, however, gums up the works by both reducing the number of LDL receptors and impairing their efficiency.

The body can make most fatty acids from carbon, hydrogen, and oxygen atoms left over from any excess fat, protein, or carbohydrate foods consumed. But three fatty acids—linoleic, arachidonic, and linolenic— cannot be made in the body and are therefore called essential fatty acids. The body needs essential fatty acids to construct healthy cell walls, make cholesterol (the body needs a certain amount of cholesterol to function normally), and make substances called prostaglandins that regulate blood pressure, blood clotting, and other functions critical to life.

How much fat do we need to be healthy? As is true with protein, much less than many people consume. Just 20 grams of dietary fat a day generally meets the body's requirement. (It is impossible, though, to enjoy a palatable diet at this fat level, so we recommend two to three times this amount each day.) Specifically, we only need to consume polyunsaturated fat, which is where essential fatty acids are found.

Most Americans consume closer to 78 grams of dietary fat per day, and much of that, unfortunately, is in the form of saturated fat. Put another way, many Americans consume about 3½ of every 10 calories as fat, when no more than 3 of every 10 is the maximum recommended. This 30 percent fat limit is essential to using Xenical successfully and minimizing side effects. It's nice to know, though, that 30 percent is also the amount recommended by official health groups for good health.

This means about 50 to 60 grams of fat daily, depending on your calorie level. While taking Xenical, you should limit the fat eaten at any one meal to just 20 grams, and snacks must be low in fat.

Dietary fat makes foods more enjoyable, but why do we get into such trouble with it? Some of the strengths of dietary fat quickly become its weaknesses. The full-bodied flavor makes it difficult to limit foods containing fat. Their caloric density, an advantage during periods of famine, also gets us into trouble quickly; just a little more of the food generally delivers a lot of calories. In addition, some of the easiest foods to grab in a hurry—fast foods and convenience foods—are often laced with lots of fat, especially saturated fat. And some foods contain fat that we can't readily see or taste, which makes it even more difficult to avoid excess fat.

Eating excess fat gets you into many health troubles. Gaining too much weight is prime among them. Unfortunately, a calorie is not a calorie as far as the body's energy-storing apparatus is concerned. Excess fat calories are stored with much greater ease and at a much lower energy cost than are excess carbohydrate calories. Whereas the body burns up 25 of every 100 extra carbohydrate calories in the process of trying to store them (as fat) for later use, it takes just 3 calories to pack away 100 extra fat calories. Put another way, fat calories are more fattening than carbohydrate calories.

In chapter 5, you'll learn how to count fat grams, whether they are part of other foods or are added fats. Learning this is key to succeeding with Xenical.

Micronutrients. So far you have learned about macronutrients, the calorie-supplying nutrients in food. We also need micronutrients, those vitamins and minerals that don't supply calories but are necessary to good health. Food scientists use the word "micro" because we need them in such small amounts, but don't let the tiny amounts fool you. They are still incredibly important to good health. Getting all the nutrients your body needs is essential to living life to the fullest. That is why we've included a summary chart of the vitamins and minerals we cannot live without. Obtaining these nutrients from food is the absolute best way. Not only is it difficult to "overdose," but you also get other benefits from food that you cannot get from a supplement. For example, nutrient-rich foods are also high in fiber and phytochemicals, plant chemicals that we know confer loads of health benefits.

The body needs all these vitamins and minerals for good health and to prevent disease. They're called essential because the body cannot make them, and so they must be harvested from a healthy diet.

Vitamins and Minerals at a Glance

Nutrient	Recommended Dietary Allowance (RDA)		Why You Need It	Problem with Getting Too Much	Foods Rich in This Nutrient
Vitamin A (Retinol)	Men:	1,000 mcg*	Essential for vision; enhances immunity; builds and maintains bone	Headache, vomiting, blurred vision, liver damage, birth defects	Liver, fish liver oil, whole milk, eggs, orange fruits, leafy green, yellow, or orange vegetables
	Women:	800 mcg			
Thiamin (B$_1$)	Men (19–50):	1.5 mg	Essential for the process that derives energy from carbohydrates, protein, and fat; essential for nerve impulses	Not toxic if taken orally	Yeast, lean pork, organ meat, legumes, seeds, nuts, unrefined cereal
	Men (over 50):	1.2 mg			
	Women (19–50):	1.1 mg			
	Women (over 50):	1 mg			
Riboflavin (B$_2$)	Men (19–50):	1.7 mg	Required for releasing energy from carbohydrates, fat, and protein; regulates hormones and helps develop red blood cells	Not toxic	Milk, yogurt, cottage cheese, meat, leafy green vegetables, whole-grain foods
	Men (over 50):	1.4 mg			
	Women (19–50):	1.3 mg			
	Women (over 50):	1.2 mg			
Niacin (B$_3$)	Men (19–50):	19 mg	Needed in the release of energy from carbohydrates; breaks down fats and proteins; helps develop red blood cells	Vascular dilation or flushing; liver injury; aggravates asthma, ulcers, and glucose intolerance associated with type 2 diabetes	Meats, fish, legumes, nuts, whole-grain foods
	Men (over 50):	15 mg			
	Women (19–50):	15 mg			
	Women (over 50):	13 mg			

Vitamins and Minerals at a Glance (continued)

Nutrient	Recommended Dietary Allowance (RDA)		Why You Need It	Problem with Getting Too Much	Foods Rich in This Nutrient
Biotin	30 to 100 mcg		Necessary for energy metabolism; makes fatty acids; breaks down amino acids	Not toxic at doses up to 10 mg	Liver, egg yolk, soybean, yeast
Pantothenic Acid	4 to 7 mg		Helps metabolize fats, carbohydrates, and protein; helps produce bile, vitamin D, red blood cells, and neurotransmitters	Doses of 10 to 20 g per day may cause diarrhea and water retention	Meats, whole-grain cereal, legumes
Vitamin B$_6$ (Pyridoxine)	Men: 2 mg	Women: 1.6 mg	Helpful in lowering blood levels of homocysteine, an amino acid associated with heart disease	Prolonged use of more than 250 mg per day can cause sensitivity to light and neurological symptoms	Chicken, fish, kidney, liver, pork, eggs
Folate (Folic Acid, Folacin)	400 mcg		Helps synthesize the DNA in rapidly growing cells; lowers homocysteine levels	At levels over 1 mg, masks the symptoms of B$_{12}$ deficiency and pernicious anemia	Yeast, liver, green and leafy vegetables, fruits

Nutrient	Recommended Amount	Function	Symptoms	Sources
Vitamin B₁₂ (Cobalamin)	2 mcg	Helps make new cells; maintains sheath around nerve fibers	No toxicity up to 100 mcg	Liver, clams, oysters, milk, seafood, eggs
Vitamin C (Ascorbic Acid)	60 mg; up to 100 mg for smokers	Antioxidant; needed for essential hormones that help regulate the body's metabolic rate during illness or stress	Nausea and diarrhea	Citrus fruits, green vegetables, peppers, tomatoes, berries, potatoes
Vitamin D	200 IU (adults 19–50) 400 IU (adults 51–70) 600 IU (adults over 70)	Promotes bone mineralization and strength by raising calcium and phosphorus levels in blood	Calcium withdrawal from bones and teeth, kidney damage, artery hardening, death	Sunlight, fish liver oil, fatty fish, egg yolk, milk
Vitamin E (Tocotrienol)	Men: 10 mg (15 IU) Women: 8 mg (12 IU)	Acts as an antioxidant	Gastrointestinal discomfort, impaired immune function	Vegetable oils, wheat germ, nuts, green leafy vegetables
Vitamin K	Men (19–24): 70 mcg Men (over 25): 80 mcg Women (19–24): 60 mcg Women (over 25): 65 mcg	Synthesizes proteins involved in blood clotting, plasma, bone, and kidneys	In newborns: anemia, high levels of bilirubin, and jaundice	Green leafy vegetables
Calcium	1,000 mg (adults 19–50) 1,200 mg (adults over 50)	Essential in bone formation and maintenance	Inhibits absorption of other minerals; kidney stones, fatigue, muscle weakness, depression, loss of appetite, nausea	Milk and dairy products, green leafy vegetables, sardines, salmon, tofu

Vitamins and Minerals at a Glance (continued)

Nutrient	Recommended Dietary Allowance (RDA)		Why You Need It	Problem with Getting Too Much	Foods Rich in This Nutrient
Iron	Men: Women (19–50): Women (over 50):	10 mg 15 mg 10 mg	Works with hemoglobin, which carries oxygen in the bloodstream	Nausea, vomiting, diarrhea, rapid heartbeat, weak pulse, dizziness, shock, confusion, death	Meat, poultry, fish, cereals, dried fruit, leafy green vegetables
Magnesium	Men: Women:	350 mg 280 mg	Works in chemical reactions that metabolize food and transmit messages between cells	Nausea, vomiting, low blood pressure, breathing difficulties, coma, heart attack	Nuts, legumes, whole grains, green vegetables, bananas
Potassium		3,500 mg	Helps transmit nerve impulses, contract muscles, maintain normal blood pressure	Muscle weakness, vomiting, cardiac arrest	Fruits, vegetables, legumes, meats
Zinc	Men: Women:	15 mg 12 mg	Necessary for growth, immune function, blood clotting, wound healing, sperm production	Lowers "good" HDL cholesterol, lowers levels of copper, shrinks red blood cells, impairs immunity	Meat, liver, eggs, seafood
Sodium		500 mg	Regulates fluid balance in body, helps in metabolism of carbohydrates and protein	Causes fluid retention and, in some people, hypertension; leaches calcium from bones	Salt, processed foods, soy sauce

* mcg = microgram = $1/1,000$ of a milligram (mg), which is $1/1,000$ of a gram (may also be written as μ g)

Now that we have learned what makes up the food we eat, let's discuss dieting.

Can Margaret Lose Weight on 1,500 Calories?

Absolutely! The problem is, most of the dieting Margarets in the world want to lose much faster. Before discussing that, let's figure out what calorie level is necessary to lose weight, using Margaret as an example.

1. Convert your body weight from pounds to kilograms by dividing by 2.2 (there are 2.2 pounds per kilogram)

   Body weight in pounds ÷ 2.2 (pounds per kilogram) = body weight in kilograms

   Margaret weighs 185 pounds: 185 pounds ÷ 2.2 pounds per kilogram = 84 kilograms

   Your calculations:

   I weigh _____ pounds: _____ pounds ÷ 2.2 pounds per kilogram = _____ kilograms

2. Determine how many calories are necessary to maintain your current body weight (not the weight you'd like to be) by multiplying your current weight by 25 calories per kilogram:

   Margaret's calculations: 84 × 25 = 2,100 calories

   Your calculations: _____ × 25 = _____ calories

3. Subtract calories to achieve enough of a calorie deficit to lose weight but not be left bingeing, hungry, or sending your body into starvation conservation. We advise subtracting 500 to 700 calories each day from the calorie level that is currently sustaining your weight.

   The range of calorie levels that Margaret can best lose weight at is created by the following calculations:

   2,100 − 500 = 1,600 calories (Margaret's upper calorie level for losing weight)

2,100 − 700 = 1,400 calories (Margaret's lower calorie level for losing weight)

As you can see, Margaret's 1,500-calorie requirement is right in the middle of her lower and higher weight loss ranges. She can, indeed, lose weight at this level.

Your calculations:

The range of calories that I can best lose weight at:

_____ − 500 = _____ calories (my upper calorie limit for losing weight)

_____ − 700 = _____ calories (my lower calorie limit for losing weight)

Watch What You Eat

Every dieter must acknowledge that there is often a discrepancy between what you think you are eating and what you are actually eating. It seems as if it's an American institution to underestimate what you are eating. It's not that we're trying to be dishonest: it's simply that we overlook some calories. But this is an easy way to pick up extra calories. Let's take a look at what happened to Don and how he picked up 706 extra calories in one day when he thought he was being conscientious.

Don forgot that he took a second helping of orange juice on the way out the door in the morning (an extra four ounces, or an extra 56 calories), didn't notice that he served himself 1 cup of rice when his meal plan called for ½ cup (an extra ½ cup of rice, or 102 calories), and neglected to weigh the roasted chicken because he thought he had become accurate at eyeballing a portion size (that cost him 93 extra calories). Standing at baseball practice that night, he didn't even realize that he was munching on the bag of chips that was being passed around, and he didn't figure the extra 455 calories into his daily calorie total at the end of the day. All told, that extra 706 calories spelled the difference between weight loss and weight maintenance for Don that day.

Adding these little calorie bundles day after day is what keeps most dieters from losing weight. These few unconscious moments help to explain why most dieters believe they are eating much less than they really are. As you'll learn in chapter 5, managing portion sizes is an extremely important part of staying on target to lose weight.

Be a Conscientious Calorie Consumer

I can't emphasize enough that you *can* lose weight while eating a reasonable number of calories. Although many dieters think they are really eating at low-calorie levels, they aren't, because of little, unconscious, but consistently frequent eating digressions. Further, because they don't realize how many calories they are eating, many people think they have to drop down to a very low level to lose weight. But taking a close look at the real-life example on these pages should give you the confidence to know that you can lose weight at a reasonable, safe, and physically and emotionally satisfying calorie level.

Xenical: Tipping the Scales in Your Favor

An example that will prove this is a typical day in Margaret's dieting life. We'll tally fat and calories as the day progresses. We're going to look at this in two ways: without Xenical and with Xenical.

Eating Without Xenical: A Tally of Calories and Fat

BREAKFAST

1 pumpkin muffin spread with 1 teaspoon margarine

1 cup skim milk

This breakfast has 264 calories and 8 grams of fat, or a total of 72 fat calories.

SNACK

1 fresh nectarine

Snack has negligible fat grams and, therefore, negligible fat calories.

LUNCH

Deli roast beef sandwich: 2 slices rye bread, 3 ounces extra-lean roast beef, mustard

Side salad: lettuce, tomatoes, sliced red onions, and favorite salad dressing on the side (using 1½ tablespoons)

Coffee

Lunch has 369 calories and 20 grams of fat, or 180 fat calories.

SNACK

2 fresh apricots or 4 halves, canned in their own juice

Snack has negligible fat grams and negligible fat calories.

DINNER

Chicken-Veggie Stir-Fry over Linguine

1 cup skim milk

1 chocolate chip cookie

Dinner has 539 calories and 16 grams of fat or 144 fat calories.

SNACK

1 apple

Orange juice spritzer: 1 cup lime seltzer plus ¼ cup orange juice

Snack has negligible fat grams and negligible fat calories.

Overall, this single day supplies a total of 1,486 calories, 90 grams protein, 25 grams fiber, and 44 grams fat (27 percent of total calories). On such a 1,500-calorie plan, Margaret should lose one to two pounds per week.

When You Hit a Plateau

Please note that with any diet plan, you will hit plateaus, or times during which weight does not budge—no matter what you do. This is normal; it represents those times when our body's metabolic machinery is adjusting to the changes it is undergoing. In a sense, the body powers down temporarily in response to your decreased calorie level. To move beyond these dispiriting plateaus, redouble your exercise efforts, continue following your nutritious diet, and have faith in your efforts to improve your health. A word of warning: don't crash-diet during these times because that will just push the body into starvation-conservation mode.

As you learned in chapter 1, Xenical helps speed weight loss by blocking the absorption of some of the dietary fat you eat. Researchers designed the drug so that it stops about 30 percent of the dietary fat at each meal (at which you take Xenical) from being absorbed. The unabsorbed portion simply passes through the body and is eliminated with the body's waste products. Let's take a look at what this means for Margaret.

Eating with Xenical: A Tally of Calories and Fat

BREAKFAST

1 pumpkin muffin spread with 1 teaspoon margarine

1 cup skim milk

This breakfast has 264 calories and 8 grams of fat, or 72 fat calories.

But with Xenical, Margaret doesn't absorb 30 percent of the 8 fat grams or 30 percent of the 72 fat calories, eliminating about 2 fat grams or 22 calories from her breakfast.

SNACK

1 fresh nectarine

This snack has negligible fat grams and, therefore, negligible fat calories.

LUNCH

Deli roast beef sandwich: 2 slices rye bread, 3 ounces extra-lean roast beef, mustard

Side salad: lettuce, tomatoes, sliced red onions, and favorite salad dressing on the side (using 2 tablespoons)

Coffee

Lunch has 369 calories and 20 grams of fat, or 180 fat calories.

With Xenical, Margaret doesn't absorb 6 grams of fat, or a total of 54 calories, removing these from her daily calorie slate.

SNACK

2 fresh apricots, or 4 halves, canned in their own juice

Snack has negligible fat grams and negligible fat calories.

DINNER

Chicken-Veggie Stir-Fry over Linguine

1 cup skim milk

1 chocolate chip cookie

Dinner has 539 calories and 16 grams of fat, or 144 fat calories.

Xenical erases about 5 grams of fat, or 43 calories, from Margaret's dinner.

SNACK

1 apple

Orange juice spritzer: 1 cup lime seltzer plus ¼ cup orange juice

Snack has negligible fat grams and negligible fat calories.

The Xenical Advantage: One Day

In just this one day, Margaret has absorbed 13 fewer grams of fat or 119 fewer calories, without exerting any extra effort.

Over the long haul, given that it takes a 3,500-calorie deficit to lose a pound, Margaret will drop one extra pound about every twenty-nine days. This depends, of course, on how many calories, and particularly how many fat calories, Margaret eats each day. In a year's time Xenical can help Margaret lose an extra thirteen pounds over and above the one or two pounds she will lose every week she follows the diet (about seven pounds per month in total). Remember, this is all possible on a calorie level that is satisfying and that won't put Margaret at risk of bingeing because she is starving at the end of the day.

Understanding all these basics, it is time for you to put the Xenical advantage to work for you. In the next chapter you'll learn exactly how and what to eat to realize this advantage. You'll start by choosing a weight goal that is good for your health and is also realistic to achieve.

4

Our Menus and Recipes

As I've said throughout this book, Xenical is intended as one part of a three-part program of weight control. It is the tool that can tip the scales in your favor—finally. The other two parts of the program are diet and exercise. In chapter 3 you learned about the principles of the Xenical diet. Here we explain the diet itself and offer four weeks of menus and recipes to get you going. Then, in chapter 5, we give you all the guidelines you will need when you're on your own—designing your own menus, counting your fat grams, creating a low-fat pantry, and eating out.

First Things First: Common Concerns and Fast Facts

Before we get to the diet, let's discuss several common concerns and important facts based on the types of questions patients asked me during the testing of Xenical.

Choosing a Weight Goal

Ideally, you should choose your weight goal by using the BMI table found on pages 38–39 of chapter 2. Find out what your weight should be for you to have a BMI of 25. This may be too ambitious a weight goal, however, and it may overwhelm you. For example, if you have fifty or more pounds to lose, you might find this so overwhelming that you decide not to tackle your weight problem at all. Here are some suggestions for working around this:

- Try setting smaller, baby-step goals. For instance, if you have fifty pounds to lose, set a goal of ten or fifteen pounds. This is far more manageable.
- Take breaks from weight loss by working on maintaining your weight for short periods and then going back to your weight-loss efforts.

Remember that weight loss research is very encouraging about smaller weight losses. Losing 5 to 10 percent of your body weight can dramatically improve your health profile, so feel good about any weight loss you achieve.

Choosing a Calorie Level

This cannot be repeated often enough: there is no reason to drop calories so low that you feel deprived. This may sound like a broken record, but if you set too low a calorie goal, you'll probably end up so hungry that you will binge. Enough said.

Using the guide found in chapter 3 (pages 63–64) for calculating your calorie needs, determine your own calorie level for losing weight. In my many years of helping people lose weight, I find a calorie level of about 1,500 is reasonable and easy to follow for an extended time. The other advantage of this calorie level is that you have an easier time getting more of the nutrients you need for good health. Nutritionists have determined that it is very difficult to get 100 percent of the Recommended Dietary Allowances for all nutrients when calorie intake drops below 1,500 (another reason weight-loss experts recommend a nutritional supplement for dieters).

The lowest calorie level I recommend for dieters is 1,300. Anything lower than that is an automatic setup for failure, not only because you get too hungry but also because the body reverts to starvation mode. In addition, lower calorie levels just aren't healthy. Yes, you are motivated to lose weight, but your good health is still critically important. When your nutrient intake drops too low, you cannot maintain a healthy immune system to fight off infections. Also, people become very fatigued at very low calorie levels and then don't have the drive to exercise.

Another word about choosing your best dieting calorie level. Younger people and men can generally lose weight at relatively high calorie levels. People who are rigorous exercisers might also want to consider dieting at the upper end of the calorie spectrum. In addition, people under a good deal of stress in their everyday lives should choose a slightly higher calorie level. Stress plus severe calorie deprivation can increase the risk of failure. It is better to eliminate this added source of stress and diet more gently. Your chances of success will be much greater.

In the real world of eating, I emphasize that dieters should also consider giving themselves the advantage of working within a range of calorie levels, as discussed below.

Being Flexible with Calorie Levels

Appetites vary day by day; some days we are hungrier than others. Some dieters have another way of thinking about this, and it often sets them up for failure. They think that if they don't stick *exactly* with the calorie level they have prescribed for themselves they have failed. Unfortunately, this dietary rigidity can lead to bingeing. If they cross over the preset diet calorie line, dieters believe they have "blown it" and then go on with reckless eating. There is a way around this, though, and it's quite easy.

Give yourself some flexibility in calorie levels to account for hungrier days. This has the psychological benefit of making you feel legal all the time, which breeds self-pride and success. Here's how to do this. Start with the lowest healthy calorie level (generally about 1,500, as advised earlier), and then give yourself a 200-calorie leeway for those hungry days. This gives you a plan for those days when appetite strikes. To encourage this method, we have created flexible menus that have several calorie levels, making it possible to slide around by 100 to 200 calories as necessary.

Why Is Fiber So High?

You will notice that our meal plans are quite high in fiber. While this is in keeping with official dietary advice to increase fiber intake for good health (fiber helps reduce the risk of some cancers and heart disease, and even helps regulate blood sugars), there is another good reason that dieters should make sure to bulk up daily. Increasing the fiber in your diet not only helps you eat fewer calories because it fills up your tummy with fewer calories. But the latest research reveals that fiber helps you lose weight by reducing the number of calories you absorb.

Fiber blocks absorption of some of the fat and protein calories you ingest, according to late-breaking research from the U.S. Department of Agriculture's Human Nutrition Research Center in Beltsville, Maryland. Researchers who studied the effect of fiber on food absorption found that each gram of fiber substituted for sugary simple carbohydrates results in a 7-calorie deficit. Translation: women who double daily fiber intake from 12 to 24 grams would absorb over 80 fewer calories each day; men who increase fiber from 18 to 36 grams daily avoid approximately 130 calories. The net result is a ten-pound weight loss in one year.

How does fiber work to negate the calories you consume? It has to do with speed—hurrying things through your digestive track, to be exact. That is also how fiber is thought to decrease the risks of cancer and heart disease. In addition to corralling fat and protein calories, fiber captures cholesterol and cancer-causing substances.

Don't be tempted to rely on a fiber supplement once per day instead of switching over to high-fiber eating. Fiber's effect of tying up extra calories relies on your eating it with each meal, and relying on supplements is often synonymous with throwing caution to the wind. Knowing you're going to satisfy your fiber needs in a supplement, it's easy to continue a low-fiber eating plan that is by nature higher in calories and fat—and fiber can negate only a limited number of calories.

Why Should I Eat Snacks?

There are two main reasons to include snacks in your daily eating plan. First, when you are limiting calories, hunger can build up. Staving off hunger pangs with regular snacks is one way to prevent bingeing. The second reason comes from fairly new research about the efficiency with which we burn larger calorie bundles as we age.

Researchers at Tufts University recently found that we may have a reduced ability to burn calories efficiently with age, especially if those calories come in big packages. The Tufts research team studied the fat-burning ability of two groups of women, one in their twenties and another that was postmenopausal. Each age group was fed three test meals of varying amounts of calories—250 calories, 500 calories, and 1,000 calories. After each test meal, the researchers measured the amount of energy each age group burned. The younger and older women had no trouble burning the 250- and 500-calorie meals, but when it came to the 1,000-calorie meal, the older women were at a big disadvantage, burning about 30 percent less fat than the younger women. In actual numbers that means the older women burned up only 187 fat calories of the large meal, while the younger ones burned up 246 calories.

Over time, people who frequently eat large meals will tend to gain weight even if they don't eat too many calories overall, say the researchers. Just eating two to three large meals per day (even if the day's total calories aren't excessive), you can gain six pounds per year.

Why does the body's "furnace" lose its efficiency? The energy-burning hormones change with age and become less effective. Insulin, the hormone "key" that unlocks the door for sugar in the blood to enter cells, becomes less efficient with age. The result: the body must make more insulin to allow the same amount of sugar into cells. This has significant consequences. Among them, an increased amount of insulin circulating in the blood causes the body to take the easy way out; rather than burn the sugar, the body stores it as fat. Once stored as fat, the body has a hard time getting rid of it. In addition, as mentioned earlier, we tend to lose muscle mass as we age. Muscle is such a powerful calorie burner that this also has the effect of turning down the body's furnace.

The solution is to divide your calories into smaller meals and snacks throughout the day, rather than just three meals. To use an analogy, just as a fire burns easier and quicker with smaller sticks than with thick logs, your body is better able to burn smaller calorie bundles. The hormones—especially insulin—work more efficiently when you feed yourself small amounts of calories at one time. As a result, your body doesn't resort to turning calories into fat.

For these important reasons you'll find at least two snacks in each day of the eating plans we've designed. If you create your own menus, divide the snack category into 3 snacks: one for midmorning, one for the afternoon, and one for the evening.

How Much Water Should I Drink, and Can I Drink Alcohol?

Drinking enough liquid is key to slimming down (and staying slimmer) for many reasons. First, drinking sufficient fluid keeps the body well hydrated, which is its natural, healthy state. I find that many times people think they are hungry when they are actually thirsty. The thirst mechanism is very intricate, but it doesn't kick in until the body is quite dehydrated. Earlier than that, though, the body does sense that something is missing, which often leads people to eat instead of drink. So, by drinking lots of water, the body stays in tune with itself. Also, the body runs more energetically when it is well hydrated. The other advantage to drinking plenty of fluids is that your stomach stays fuller, which also helps you eat less.

But what about alcohol and other types of beverages? Here are some general guidelines that should be helpful when you choose things to drink:

- Alcohol. If you want to drink alcohol, remember that it contains quite a lot of calories. The easiest way to account for it is to use grain food servings for the alcohol calories you spend. Four ounces of wine, 1 ounce of hard liquor, or 12 ounces of light beer count for one grain food serving. One regular beer would use up two grain food servings. Note that if you use a mixer, it can also contain calories. Look for low-calorie options where possible. And do check with your physician about the use of alcohol, especially on a regular basis.

- Soda, lemonade, and other calorie-containing beverages. The calories in these beverages can wreak havoc with anyone's waist line. For one, we often drink these things when we are really thirsty, which means we down eight to sixteen ounces quite quickly—without even thinking about it. Also, these calories are empty—or don't contain any useful nutrients with their calories. My advice is to choose the low-calorie versions of these drinks.
- Juices. Orange juice seems to define breakfast in America. While you are on a lower calorie eating plan, however, you might want to consider eating the whole fruit, rather than drinking the juice. The whole orange, for example, is far more filling than the four ounces of juice you get for the same number of calories (yes, that's a small glass of juice). Ditto for apple juice vs. the whole apple.
- Coffee and tea. The other beverages that define breakfast in America, and most other meals and breaks, are coffee and tea. While these drinks, if they contain caffeine, will not help to hydrate your body—the caffeine acts as a diuretic, causing your body to lose the fluid as fast as you drink it—they do not appear to be harmful if consumed in moderation. However, there are a few instances when you need to be wary of the calories these types of drinks can bring along with them. If you regularly consume milk-based coffee drinks such as lattes and cappuccinos, be aware of the fat in the full-cream milk. Ask for a "skinny-chino" and lattes made with fat-free milk. Many of the commercially prepared iced teas on the market are as high in sugar as sodas are. As with the sodas, look for the low-calorie versions where possible.
- Plain old water. This is still your best bet. Make it cold, make it tart with lemons and limes, or drink it with fizz (seltzer or mineral water) if you want to.
- Aim to enjoy at least sixty-four ounces of hydrating fluids each day. This can include any drink that does not contain alcohol or caffeine. In other words, water, juice, and noncaffeinated soda all count toward your daily fluid intake. To gauge whether or not you are drinking enough, find a glass that holds eight ounces and be sure to fill it eight times each day.

How to Use Our Menus

Our weight-loss menus allow you 1,300 calories at the low end and 1,700 calories at the high end. The five calorie levels mean that this diet is not the familiar "one size fits all" variety. You can tailor it to the level of calorie intake that is right for you. Read through the following example of one day from the program to learn exactly how to use it. We've created these meal plans and recipes especially for use with Xenical, which makes following this diet a snap. You will find four weeks of these menus, accompanied by a multitude of tempting recipes that will show you just how tasty healthy eating can be. Some of these delicious, nutritious recipes come from Larry Forgione, talented chef and proprietor of well-known restaurants, including An American Place in Manhattan.

First, note the foods you'll need for the day. Next choose the calorie level you want to follow from the top row. Then note the portion sizes for that calorie level in the column under that amount. Read the additional notes about portion sizes later in this chapter. Briefly, though, you'll see that the difference between calorie levels is totally dependent on portion size. You'll notice that in some cases, foods are eliminated to accommodate the lower calorie levels; these are indicated by the word "omit."

Food	1,300 calories	1,400 calories	1,500 calories	1,600 calories	1,700 calories
BREAKFAST					
Low-fat extra calcium cottage cheese	¹/₂ cup	¹/₂ cup	¹/₂ cup	¹/₂ cup	¹/₂ cup
Sliced strawberries	1 cup	1 cup	1 cup	1 cup	1 cup
Whole wheat English muffin	¹/₂	¹/₂	¹/₂	1	1
Light tub margarine	2 teaspoons	2 teaspoons	2 teaspoons	2 teaspoons	2 teaspoons
MORNING SNACK					
Nectarine	1	1	1	1	1

Food	1,300 calories	1,400 calories	1,500 calories	1,600 calories	1,700 calories
LUNCH					
Fresh Garden Salad with Balsamic Vinaigrette	Recipe as shown	Recipe as shown	Recipe as shown	Recipe as shown	Use ¾ cup garbanzo beans
Whole wheat crackers	6	6	6	6	6

All menu items in italics and shaded signify a recipe that you'll find in this chapter following the menu plans. We've divided the recipes into categories: breakfast, lunch, dinner, and dessert. In most cases you'll simply prepare the recipe as indicated and then serve the required portion size, which we've indicated with the phrase "recipe as shown." To accommodate the various calorie levels, though, we've occasionally indicated how you should modify the recipe. For example, you'd prepare the Fresh Garden Salad with Balsamic Vinaigrette as indicated in the recipe but then add an extra ¼ cup of garbanzo beans if you are aiming for the 1,700-calorie level.

AFTERNOON SNACK

Bok choy	Omit	2 stalks	2 stalks	2 stalks	2 stalks
Fat-free cream cheese	Omit	4 teaspoons	4 teaspoons	4 teaspoons	4 teaspoons
Raisins	Omit	4 tablespoons	4 tablespoons	4 tablespoons	4 tablespoons
Air-popped popcorn	I cup	Omit	Omit	Omit	Omit
Lime seltzer	2 cups	2 cups	2 cups	2 cups	2 cups

The snacks for this day illustrate an important feature in our menus. Sometimes it is necessary to substitute some foods for others to achieve the desired calorie levels. This is especially true when meeting the lower calorie requirements. Here, for instance, the lower calorie level accommodates a very low calorie snack such as popcorn, while the higher dieting levels allow more interesting snacks such as bok choy topped with fat-free cream cheese and raisins—a fabulously delicious snack, by the way!

Food	1,300 calories	1,400 calories	1,500 calories	1,600 calories	1,700 calories
			DINNER		
Grilled salmon	3 ounces	3 ounces	3 ounces	3 ounces	4 ounces
Sour Cream and Chives Baked Potato	Recipe as shown	Recipe as shown	Recipe as shown	Use 2 tablespoons low-fat sour cream	Use 2 tablespoons low-fat sour cream
Asparagus spears with freshly squeezed lemon	6	6	6	6	6
Light tub margarine	I teaspoon	I teaspoon	I teaspoon	I teaspoon	I teaspoon
Skim milk	Omit	I cup	I cup	I cup	I cup
			EVENING SNACK		
Nonfat frozen yogurt	$^1/_2$ cup	$^1/_2$ cup	$^1/_2$ cup	$^1/_2$ cup	$^1/_2$ cup
			DAILY NUTRITION TOTALS		
Calories	1,327	1,412	1,497	1,604	1,667
Fat (g)	42	42	40	43	42
Carbohydrates (g)	185	197	225	241	251
Protein (g)	68	77	79	83	91
Fiber (g)	31	31	33	35	38
Cals. from fat (%)	27	26	23	23	22

This final box gives you the specifics on what you've eaten. We've included information on protein, carbohydrate, fiber, and fat grams, as well as the percentage of calories you've eaten as fat, just for the sake of completeness. Note that each meal and each day contain no more than 30 percent of calories as fat, which is one of the most important features of the Xenical eating style.

Controlling Portion Sizes: Tips and Hints

Portion control is one of the most challenging aspects of weight control but also one of the most important keys to success. Choosing food wisely is almost useless if portions are too generous. Let's look at one real example. If you plan to eat three ounces of grilled salmon for dinner with 1 cup of wild rice (and lots of veggies, of course), but instead serve five ounces of salmon and 1¼ cups of wild rice, you eat 145 extra calories. Even these seemingly small infractions will result in gaining an extra pound every twenty-four days, all other things being equal.

Measure carefully for at least one week; this will help you learn portion sizes. After that, monitor your ability to estimate portion size by measuring on one specified day of each week. There is another secret: rather than use serving spoons, use measuring cups and measuring spoons. Once you make this transition, it just becomes a way of life. Another trick is to measure the capacity of the dishes and cups you use, and then use the same ones consistently. If your cereal bowls hold two cups, for example, you'll know that you should fill the bowl half full if you are having one cup of cereal. Find the drinking glass that holds eight ounces and use it consistently.

A Visual Guide to Serving Size

Food	Number of Servings	Visual
I cup cooked rice or pasta	2 grain food	tennis ball
I slice bread	I grain food	compact disk case
I cup raw vegetables or fruit	I fruit or vegetable	tennis ball
1/2 cup cooked vegetables or fruit	I fruit or vegetable	small fist
I ounce cheese	I high-fat protein	pair of dice
I teaspoon olive oil	I fat	half-dollar
3 ounces cooked meat	3 protein	deck of cards or cassette tape

Menus

	WEEK ONE				
	Week One, Day One				
Food	1,300 calories	1,400 calories	1,500 calories	1,600 calories	1,700 calories
	BREAKFAST				
Strawberry-Banana-Kiwi Breakfast Smoothie	Use 1/2 banana; omit wheat germ	Use 1/2 banana; omit wheat germ	Use 1/2 banana; omit wheat germ	Recipe as shown	Recipe as shown
	MORNING SNACK				
Whole wheat bagel	1/2	1/2	1/2	1/2	I
Fat-free cream cheese	I tablespoon	I tablespoon	I tablespoon	I tablespoon	I tablespoon

Food	1,300 calories	1,400 calories	1,500 calories	1,600 calories	1,700 calories
LUNCH					
Tuna Fish on Pita	Recipe as shown	Recipe as shown	Recipe as shown	Recipe as shown	Recipe as shown
Skim milk	¹/₂ cup	¹/₂ cup	I cup	I cup	I cup
Chocolate chip cookie	Omit	Omit	I	I	I
AFTERNOON SNACK					
Fresh peach	I	I	I	I	I
Skim milk	Omit	¹/₂ cup	¹/₂ cup	¹/₂ cup	¹/₂ cup
DINNER					
Grilled skinless, boneless chicken breast	3 ounces	3 ounces	3 ounces	3 ounces	3 ounces
Brown rice	¹/₂ cup	¹/₂ cup	¹/₂ cup	¹/₂ cup	¹/₂ cup
Skim milk	¹/₂ cup	I cup	I cup	I cup	I cup
Grilled Vegetable Medley	Recipe as shown	Recipe as shown	Recipe as shown	Recipe as shown	Recipe as shown
EVENING SNACK					
Extra-calcium orange juice	¹/₂ cup	¹/₂ cup	¹/₂ cup	¹/₂ cup	¹/₂ cup
NUTRITION TOTALS FOR DAY ONE					
Calories	1,315	1,401	1,485	1,618	1,691
Fat (g)	36	36	38	42	42
Carbohydrates (g)	182	194	210	230	246
Protein (g)	75	84	87	92	95
Fiber (g)	25	25	26	29	32
Cals. from fat (%)	24	23	22	22	22

Week One, Day Two

Food	1,300 calories	1,400 calories	1,500 calories	1,600 calories	1,700 calories
BREAKFAST					
Low-fat extra-calcium cottage cheese	¹/₂ cup	¹/₂ cup	¹/₂ cup	¹/₂ cup	¹/₂ cup
Sliced strawberries	I cup	I cup	I cup	I cup	I cup
Whole wheat English muffin	¹/₂	¹/₂	¹/₂	I	I
Light tub margarine	2 teaspoons	2 teaspoons	2 teaspoons	2 teaspoons	2 teaspoons

Food	1,300 calories	1,400 calories	1,500 calories	1,600 calories	1,700 calories
			Week One, Day Two (continued)		

MORNING SNACK

Food	1,300 calories	1,400 calories	1,500 calories	1,600 calories	1,700 calories
Nectarine	1	1	1	1	1

LUNCH

Fresh Garden Salad with Balsamic Vinaigrette	Recipe as shown	Recipe as shown	Recipe as shown	Recipe as shown	Use ³/₄ cup garbanzo beans
Whole wheat crackers	6	6	6	6	6

AFTERNOON SNACK

Bok choy	Omit	2 stalks	2 stalks	2 stalks	2 stalks
Fat-free cream cheese	Omit	4 teaspoons	4 teaspoons	4 teaspoons	4 teaspoons
Raisins	Omit	4 tablespoons	4 tablespoons	4 tablespoons	4 tablespoons
Air-popped popcorn	1 cup	Omit	Omit	Omit	Omit
Lime seltzer	2 cups	2 cups	2 cups	2 cups	2 cups

DINNER

Grilled salmon	3 ounces	3 ounces	3 ounces	3 ounces	4 ounces
Sour Cream and Chives Baked Potato	Recipe as shown	Recipe as shown	Recipe as shown	Use 2 tablespoons low-fat sour cream	Use 2 tablepoons low-fat sour cream
Asparagus spears with fresh lemon juice	6	6	6	6	6
Light tub margarine	1 teaspoon	1 teaspoon	1 teaspoon	1 teaspoon	1 teaspoon
Skim milk	Omit	1 cup	1 cup	1 cup	1 cup

EVENING SNACK

Nonfat frozen yogurt	¹/₂ cup	¹/₂ cup	¹/₂ cup	¹/₂ cup	¹/₂ cup

NUTRITION TOTALS FOR DAY TWO

Calories	1,327	1,412	1,497	1,604	1,667
Fat (g)	42	42	40	43	42
Carbohydrates (g)	185	197	225	241	251
Protein (g)	68	77	79	83	91
Fiber (g)	31	31	33	35	38
Cals. from fat (%)	27	26	23	23	22

	1,300 calories	1,400 calories	1,500 calories	1,600 calories	1,700 calories
			Week One, Day Three		
Food	1,300 calories	1,400 calories	1,500 calories	1,600 calories	1,700 calories
BREAKFAST					
Peanut Butter and Banana Breakfast Smoothie	Recipe as shown	Recipe as shown	Recipe as shown	Recipe as shown	Recipe as shown
MORNING SNACK					
Apple	1	1	1	1	1
LUNCH					
Lean Turkey Sandwich on Whole Wheat	Use 1 slice whole wheat bread	Use 1 slice whole wheat bread	Use 1 slice whole wheat bread	Recipe as shown	Recipe as shown
Skim milk	1 cup	1 cup	1 cup	1 cup	1 cup
Orange	1	1	1	1	1
AFTERNOON SNACK					
Nonfat fig bar	1	1	1	1	2
Skim milk	1/2 cup	1/2 cup	1/2 cup	1/2 cup	1/2 cup
DINNER					
Lemon, Basil, and Ginger Tofu Stir-Fry with Spinach Rotini	Use 1/2 cup pasta	Use 1/2 cup pasta	Recipe as shown	Recipe as shown	Recipe as shown
Skim milk	1/2 cup	1/2 cup	1/2 cup	1/2 cup	1/2 cup
EVENING SNACK					
Low-fat micro-wave popcorn	1 cup	3 cups	3 cups	3 cups	3 cups
Extra-calcium orange juice	Omit	1/2 cup	1/2 cup	1/2 cup	1/2 cup
NUTRITION TOTALS FOR DAY THREE					
Calories	1,359	1,457	1,556	1,625	1,692
Fat (g)	40	42	43	43	43
Carbohydrates (g)	204	244	244	257	272
Protein (g)	63	65	68	71	72
Fiber (g)	27	32	33	35	35
Cals. from fat (%)	25	24	23	23	22

	Week One, Day Four				
Food	1,300 calories	1,400 calories	1,500 calories	1,600 calories	1,700 calories
	BREAKFAST				
Oatmeal with Apple and Brown Sugar	Recipe as shown	Recipe as shown	Recipe as shown	Recipe as shown	Recipe as shown
	MORNING SNACK				
Sliced Strawberries	¹/₂ cup	¹/₂ cup	¹/₂ cup	¹/₂ cup	¹/₂ cup
	LUNCH				
Spicy Bean Tortilla	Use small tortilla	Use small tortilla	Recipe as shown	Recipe as shown	Recipe as shown
Nectarine	1	1	1	1	1
Iced tea	2 cups	2 cups	2 cups	2 cups	2 cups
	AFTERNOON SNACK				
Blueberries	¹/₂ cup	¹/₂ cup	¹/₂ cup	¹/₂ cup	¹/₂ cup
Skim milk	Omit	Omit	¹/₂ cup	¹/₂ cup	¹/₂ cup
	DINNER				
Juicy Grilled Hamburger with Vidalia Onion on Whole Wheat Bun	Recipe as shown	Recipe as shown	Recipe as shown	Recipe as shown	Recipe as shown
Steamed broccoli	1 cup	1 cup	1 cup	1 cup	1 cup
Light tub margarine	1 tablespoon	1 tablespoon	1 tablespoon	2 tablespoons	2 tablespoons
Skim milk	Omit	Omit	1 cup	1 cup	1 cup
Mint iced tea	2 cups	2 cups	Omit	Omit	Omit
	EVENING SNACK				
Nonfat frozen yogurt	Omit	Omit	Omit	¹/₂ cup	1 cup
Sliced strawberries	¹/₂ cup	¹/₂ cup	¹/₂ cup	¹/₂ cup	¹/₂ cup
Low-fat whipped topping	2 tablespoons	2 tablespoons	2 tablespoons	Omit	Omit

Food	1,300 calories	1,400 calories	1,500 calories	1,600 calories	1,700 calories
NUTRITION TOTALS FOR DAY FOUR					
Calories	1,289	1,375	1,443	1,573	1,669
Fat (g)	35	36	43	43	43
Carbohydrates (g)	187	198	208	224	243
Protein (g)	69	77	82	87	91
Fiber (g)	30	30	30	30	30
Cals. from fat (%)	24	22	24	24	22

Week One, Day Five

Food	1,300 calories	1,400 calories	1,500 calories	1,600 calories	1,700 calories
BREAKFAST					
Western Omelet	Recipe as shown	Recipe as shown	Recipe as shown	Recipe as shown	Recipe as shown
Whole wheat toast	1 slice	1 slice	1 slice	1 slice	1 slice
Light tub margarine	1 teaspoon	1 teaspoon	1 teaspoon	1 teaspoon	2 teaspoons
MORNING SNACK					
Watermelon cubes	1 cup	1 cup	1 cup	1 cup	1 cup
LUNCH					
Ham Sandwich on Rye	Use 1 slice rye bread; substitute mustard for mayonnaise	Use 1 slice rye bread; substitute mustard for mayonnaise	Recipe as shown	Recipe as shown	Recipe as shown
Skim milk	Substitute seltzer	1 cup	1 cup	1 cup	1 cup
AFTERNOON SNACK					
Cantaloupe cubes	1 cup	1 cup	1 cup	1 cup	1 cup
DINNER					
Chicken Stir-Fry	Recipe as shown	Recipe as shown	Recipe as shown	Recipe as shown	Recipe as shown
Brown rice	1/2 cup	1/2 cup	1/2 cup	1/2 cup	1/2 cup
Raspberry Cheesecake	Recipe as shown	Recipe as shown	Recipe as shown	Recipe as shown	Recipe as shown

Week One, Day Five (continued)

Food	1,300 calories	1,400 calories	1,500 calories	1,600 calories	1,700 calories
EVENING SNACK					
Sliced strawberries	¹/₂ cup	¹/₂ cup	¹/₂ cup	¹/₂ cup	¹/₂ cup
Nonfat frozen yogurt	Omit	Omit	Omit	¹/₂ cup	I cup
NUTRITION TOTALS FOR DAY FIVE					
Calories	1,315	1,401	1,505	1,600	1,712
Fat (g)	42	42	46	46	49
Carbohydrates (g)	158	170	185	204	223
Protein (g)	85	93	96	101	105
Fiber (g)	20	20	21	21	21
Cals. from fat (%)	28	27	27	25	25

Week One, Day Six

Food	1,300 calories	1,400 calories	1,500 calories	1,600 calories	1,700 calories
BREAKFAST					
Whole-grain bagel	I	I	I	I	I
Part-skim mozzarella cheese	I ounce	2 ounces	2 ounces	2 ounces	2 ounces
Extra-calcium orange juice	¹/₂ cup	¹/₂ cup	¹/₂ cup	I cup	I cup
MORNING SNACK					
Nonfat fruited yogurt	¹/₂ cup	¹/₂ cup	¹/₂ cup	¹/₂ cup	¹/₂ cup
LUNCH					
Watercress Black Bean Salad	Recipe as shown	Recipe as shown	Recipe as shown	Recipe as shown	Use 3 tablespoons regular Italian salad dressing
Whole wheat crackers	5	5	5	5	8
Ice water with lemon wedge	2 cups or more	2 cups or more	2 cups or more	2 cups or more	2 cups or more

Food	1,300 calories	1,400 calories	1,500 calories	1,600 calories	1,700 calories
	AFTERNOON SNACK				
Skim milk	1 cup	1 cup	1 cup	1 cup	1 cup
Carrot sticks	1 carrot	1 carrot	1 carrot	1 carrot	1 carrot
Fat-free ranch dressing or dip	2 tablespoons	2 tablespoons	2 tablespoons	2 tablespoons	2 tablespoons
	DINNER				
Broiled fillet of sole	4 ounces	4 ounces	4 ounces	4 ounces	4 ounces
Small sweet potato	1	1	1	1	1
Brown sugar (for sweet potato)	1 teaspoon	1 teaspoon	1 teaspoon	1 teaspoon	1 teaspoon
Asparagus spears with fresh lemon juice	6	6	6	6	6
Light tub margarine (for sweet potato and asparagus)	4 teaspoons	4 teaspoons	4 teaspoons	4 teaspoons	4 teaspoons
Skim milk	1/2 cup	1/2 cup	1/2 cup	1/2 cup	1/2 cup
	EVENING SNACK				
Cantaloupe cubes	Omit	Omit	1 cup	1 cup	1 cup
Sliced strawberries	1 cup	1 cup	1 cup	1 cup	1 cup
Blueberries	1/2 cup	1/2 cup	1/2 cup	1/2 cup	1/2 cup
Vanilla nonfat yogurt	Omit	Omit	1/4 cup	1/4 cup	1/4 cup
	NUTRITION TOTALS FOR DAY SIX				
Calories	1,335	1,415	1,523	1,573	1,695
Fat (g)	39	44	45	45	55
Carbohydrates (g)	184	185	207	218	228
Protein (g)	78	86	91	91	92
Fiber (g)	35	35	37	41	42
Cals. from fat (%)	25	27	25	25	28

Food	1,300 calories	1,400 calories	1,500 calories	1,600 calories	1,700 calories
			Week One, Day Seven		
BREAKFAST					
Raspberry-Vanilla Smoothie	Change to 1/2 cup raspberries	Recipe as shown	Recipe as shown	Recipe as shown	Recipe as shown
MORNING SNACK					
Fresh peach	1	1	1	1	1
LUNCH					
Spinach-Lentil Salad	Use 1 tablespoon olive oil	Recipe as shown	Recipe as shown	Recipe as shown	Use 3 tablespoons olive oil
Whole wheat crackers plus 1 tablespoon light margarine	4 crackers	4 crackers	4 crackers	4 crackers	5 crackers
Skim milk	1 cup	1 cup	1 cup	1 cup	1 cup
AFTERNOON SNACK					
Apple	Omit	Omit	1/2	1	1
DINNER					
Roasted Red Pepper, Salmon, and Quinoa Salad	Recipe as shown	Recipe as shown	Recipe as shown	Recipe as shown	Recipe as shown
Skim milk	Omit	Omit	Omit	1/2 cup	1/2 cup
EVENING SNACK					
Fresh orange	1	1	1	1	1
NUTRITION TOTALS FOR DAY SEVEN					
Calories	1,333	1,452	1,493	1,626	1,693
Fat (g)	35	48	49	55	58
Carbohydrates (g)	195	195	206	222	232
Protein (g)	70	70	70	74	75
Fiber (g)	39	39	41	42	47
Cals. from fat (%)	23	29	28	29	30

	WEEK TWO				
	Week Two, Day One				
Food	*1,300 calories*	*1,400 calories*	*1,500 calories*	*1,600 calories*	*1,700 calories*
BREAKFAST					
Oat bran bagel	¹/₂	¹/₂	¹/₂	¹/₂	¹/₂
Peanut butter	4 teaspoons	4 teaspoons	4 teaspoons	4 teaspoons	4 teaspoons
Favorite jam	Omit	Omit	Omit	Omit	1 tablespoon
Skim milk	1 cup	1 cup	1 cup	1 cup	1 cup
MORNING SNACK					
Hot chamomile tea	2 cups	2 cups	2 cups	2 cups	2 cups
LUNCH					
Cheesy Veggie Pile	Use 1 slice American cheese; use 1 tablespoon low-fat mayonnaise	Use 1 tablespoon low-fat mayonnaise	Use 1 tablespoon low-fat mayonnaise	Recipe as shown	Recipe as shown
Apple	Omit	Omit	Omit	Omit	1
Lime seltzer	2 cups	2 cups	2 cups	2 cups	2 cups
AFTERNOON SNACK					
Sliced peach	1	1	1	1	1
Fat-free Cool Whip	Omit	Omit	Omit	2 tablespoons	2 tablespoons
DINNER					
Black Bean, Barley, and Leek Soup	Recipe as shown	Recipe as shown	Recipe as shown	Recipe as shown	Recipe as shown
Whole wheat crackers	3	5	5	5	5
Low-fat cream cheese	1 tablespoon	1 tablespoon	1 tablespoon	1 tablespoon	1 tablespoon
Skim milk	Omit	Omit	1 cup	1 cup	1 cup
Mint iced tea	2 cups	2 cups	Omit	Omit	Omit

	1,300 calories	1,400 calories	1,500 calories	1,600 calories	1,700 calories
	Week Two, Day One (continued)				
Food					
EVENING SNACK					
Lemon-Mint Banana-Blueberry Fruit Salad	Omit banana	Use ½ banana	Use ½ banana	Recipe as shown	Recipe as shown
NUTRITION TOTALS FOR DAY ONE					
Calories	1,261	1,429	1,515	1,624	1,711
Fat (g)	43	52	52	54	56
Carbohydrates (g)	180	200	212	232	260
Protein (g)	51	57	65	66	62
Fiber (g)	33	35	35	37	40
Cals. from fat (%)	30	30	30	29	28

	1,300 calories	1,400 calories	1,500 calories	1,600 calories	1,700 calories
	Week Two, Day Two				
Food					
BREAKFAST					
Peanut Butter and Banana Breakfast Smoothie	Recipe as shown	Recipe as shown	Recipe as shown	Recipe as shown	Recipe as shown
MORNING SNACK					
Fat-free fig bar	Omit	1	1	1	1
Skim milk	½ cup	½ cup	½ cup	½ cup	½ cup
LUNCH					
Mandarin Orange Broil	Recipe as shown	Recipe as shown	Recipe as shown	Increase to whole English muffin	Increase to whole English muffin
Carrot-Broccoli-Lemon Salad	Recipe as shown	Recipe as shown	Recipe as shown	Recipe as shown	Recipe as shown

Food	1,300 calories	1,400 calories	1,500 calories	1,600 calories	1,700 calories
AFTERNOON SNACK					
Low-sodium vegetable juice	I cup	I cup	I cup	I cup	I cup
Red grapes	Omit	Omit	Omit	¹/₂ cup	I cup
DINNER					
Hearty Chicken Tabbouleh Salad	Recipe as shown	Recipe as shown	Recipe as shown	Recipe as shown	Recipe as shown
Mint iced tea	2 cups	2 cups	Omit	Omit	Omit
Skim milk	Omit	Omit	I cup	I cup	I cup
EVENING SNACK					
Medium fresh orange	I	I	I	I	I
NUTRITION TOTALS FOR DAY TWO					
Calories	1,306	1,374	1,460	1,584	1,695
Fat (g)	44	44	44	45	46
Carbohydrates (g)	167	183	195	222	250
Protein (g)	73	74	82	85	86
Fiber (g)	29	29	29	30	32
Cals. from fat (%)	29	28	26	25	24

	Week Two, Day Three				
Food	1,300 calories	1,400 calories	1,500 calories	1,600 calories	1,700 calories
BREAKFAST					
Green Pepper Omelet	Prepare with I egg	Prepare with I egg	Recipe as shown	Recipe as shown	Recipe as shown
Whole wheat toast	I slice	I slice	I slice	I slice	I slice
Light tub margarine	I tablespoon	I tablespoon	I tablespoon	I tablespoon	I tablespoon
Skim milk	¹/₂ cup	I cup	I cup	I cup	I cup
MORNING SNACK					
Red grapes	¹/₂ cup	¹/₂ cup	¹/₂ cup	¹/₂ cup	¹/₂ cup

			Week Two, Day Three (continued)		
Food	1,300 calories	1,400 calories	1,500 calories	1,600 calories	1,700 calories
LUNCH					
Tomato Turkey Stack	Recipe as shown	Recipe as shown	Increase turkey to 3 ounces	Increase turkey to 3 ounces	Increase turkey to 3 ounces
Sweet Pepper Medley	Recipe as shown	Recipe as shown	Recipe as shown	Recipe as shown	Recipe as shown
Raspberry-flavored seltzer	As desired	As desired	As desired	As desired	As desired
AFTERNOON SNACK					
Fresh orange	1	1	1	1	1
Oat bran pretzels	Omit	Omit	Omit	Omit	1 ounce
DINNER					
Rosemary Roasted Winter Veggies and Chicken	1/4 recipe	1/4 recipe	1/4 recipe	1/4 recipe	1/4 recipe
Hot tea with lemon	As desired	As desired	As desired	As desired	As desired
Skim milk	Omit	Omit	Omit	1 cup	1 cup
EVENING SNACK					
Caffè latte: 1/2 cup favorite flavored coffee plus 1/2 cup hot milk; artificial sweetener as desired	1 serving	1 serving	1 serving	1 serving	1 serving
Fig bar	Omit	1	1	1	1
NUTRITION TOTALS FOR DAY THREE					
Calories	1,305	1,413	1,510	1,596	1,709
Fat (g)	43	44	49	49	51
Carbohydrates (g)	177	198	199	211	233
Protein (g)	67	71	84	92	95
Fiber (g)	29	29	29	29	31
Cals. from fat (%)	29	27	28	27	26

Food	1,300 calories	1,400 calories	1,500 calories	1,600 calories	1,700 calories
Week Two, Day Four					
BREAKFAST					
Banana Almond Oatmeal	Recipe as shown	Recipe as shown	Recipe as shown	Recipe as shown plus I additional tablespoon slivered almonds	Recipe as shown plus I additional tablespoon slivered almonds
MORNING SNACK					
Large fresh nectarine	I	I	I	I	I
LUNCH					
Tuna Tomato Stack	Omit I slice of bread	Recipe as shown	Recipe as shown	Recipe as shown	Recipe as shown
Large fresh orange	Omit	I	I	I	I
Skim milk	Omit	Omit	Omit	Omit	I cup
AFTERNOON SNACK					
Air-popped popcorn	Omit	Omit	I cup	I cup	I cup
Extra-calcium orange juice	¹/₂ cup	¹/₂ cup	¹/₂ cup	¹/₂ cup	¹/₂ cup
DINNER					
Turkey Burger on Bun with Sliced Vidalia Onion	Recipe as shown	Recipe as shown	Recipe as shown	Recipe as shown	Recipe as shown
Steamed Veggies with Basil and Olive Oil	Recipe as shown	Recipe as shown	Recipe as shown	Recipe as shown	Recipe as shown
Skim milk	¹/₂ cup	¹/₂ cup	¹/₂ cup	I cup	I cup
EVENING SNACK					
Low-fat vanilla yogurt	¹/₄ cup	¹/₄ cup	¹/₂ cup	¹/₂ cup	¹/₂ cup
Fresh sliced strawberries	¹/₂ cup	¹/₂ cup	¹/₂ cup	¹/₂ cup	¹/₂ cup

Week Two, Day Four (continued)

NUTRITION TOTALS FOR DAY FOUR

Calories	1,302	1,432	1,515	1,597	1,731
Fat (g)	42	43	44	48	48
Carbohydrates (g)	164	193	207	215	227
Protein (g)	78	82	86	91	110
Fiber (g)	22	27	28	29	29
Cals. from fat (%)	28	26	25	26	24

Week Two, Day Five

Food	1,300 calories	1,400 calories	1,500 calories	1,600 calories	1,700 calories
BREAKFAST					
Oat bran bagel	1/2	1/2	1	1	1
Peanut butter	1 tablespoon	2 tablespoons	2 tablespoons	3 tablespoons	3 tablespoons
Coffee	As desired	As desired	As desired	As desired	As desired
MORNING SNACK					
Skim milk	1 cup	1 cup	1 cup	1 cup	1 cup
LUNCH					
Confetti Rice Salad	Recipe as shown	Recipe as shown	Recipe as shown	Recipe as shown	Recipe as shown
Hot herbal tea	As desired	As desired	As desired	As desired	As desired
AFTERNOON SNACK					
Mint iced tea	As desired	As desired	As desired	As desired	As desired
DINNER					
Soy-Orange Marinated Red Snapper	Recipe as shown	Recipe as shown	Recipe as shown	Recipe as shown	Recipe as shown
Baked potato	1 small	1 small	1 small	1 small	1 small
Light margarine	1 tablespoon	1 tablespoon	1 tablespoon	1 tablespoon	1 tablespoon
Steamed spinach with lemon juice	1 cup	1 cup	1 cup	1 cup	1 cup
Skim milk	1/2 cup	1/2 cup	1/2 cup	1/2 cup	1/2 cup

Food	1,300 calories	1,400 calories	1,500 calories	1,600 calories	1,700 calories
EVENING SNACK					
Fresh raspberries	¹/₂ cup	¹/₂ cup	¹/₂ cup	¹/₂ cup	¹/₂ cup
Low-fat frozen dairy topping	Omit	Omit	Omit	Omit	2 tablespoons
NUTRITION TOTALS FOR DAY FIVE					
Calories	1,300	1,394	1,534	1,629	1,679
Fat (g)	35	43	43	51	52
Carbohydrates (g)	179	183	212	215	224
Protein (g)	77	81	86	90	91
Fiber (g)	33	34	36	37	41
Cals. from fat (%)	23	27	25	27	27

Week Two, Day Six

Food	1,300 calories	1,400 calories	1,500 calories	1,600 calories	1,700 calories
BREAKFAST					
Breakfast Peanut Fruit Salad	Decrease yogurt to ¹/₂ cup	Recipe as shown	Recipe as shown	Recipe as shown	Add additional ¹/₂ banana and additional 1 tablespoon peanuts
Hot tea	As desired	As desired	As desired	As desired	As desired
MORNING SNACK					
Trail mix: raisins and dried cranberries	2 tablespoons each fruit	2 tablespoons each fruit	2 tablespoons each fruit	2 tablespoons each fruit	2 tablespoons each fruit
Hot herbal tea	As desired	As desired	As desired	As desired	As desired
LUNCH					
Black Bean Salad	Recipe as shown	Recipe as shown	Recipe as shown	Recipe as shown	Recipe as shown
Bagel chips	Omit	Omit	¹/₂ ounce	1 ounce	1 ounce
Iced seltzer water	As desired	As desired	As desired	As desired	As desired
AFTERNOON SNACK					
Fresh tangerine	1	1	1	1	1

Week Two, Day Six (continued)

Food	1,300 calories	1,400 calories	1,500 calories	1,600 calories	1,700 calories
DINNER					
Creamed Chicken on Toast	1/4 recipe	1/4 recipe	1/4 recipe	1/4 recipe	1/4 recipe
Steamed spinach tossed with lemon juice and 1 teaspoon extra-virgin olive oil	1 cup	1 cup	1 cup	1 cup	1 cup
Skim milk	Omit	Omit	1/2 cup	1/2 cup	1/2 cup
EVENING SNACK					
Lime seltzer water	As desired	As desired	As desired	As desired	As desired
NUTRITION TOTALS FOR DAY SIX					
Calories	1,324	1,429	1,532	1,592	1,695
Fat (g)	43	45	47	48	53
Carbohydrates (g)	178	195	212	222	238
Protein (g)	74	80	85	86	89
Fiber (g)	35	36	36	38	40
Cals. from fat (%)	28	27	26	26	27

Week Two, Day Seven

Food	1,300 calories	1,400 calories	1,500 calories	1,600 calories	1,700 calories
BREAKFAST					
The Moistest Pumpkin Muffins	1	1	1	2	2
Hot herbal tea	As desired	As desired	As desired	As desired	As desired
MORNING SNACK					
Skim milk	1/2 cup	1/2 cup	1 cup	1 cup	1 cup

Food	1,300 calories	1,400 calories	1,500 calories	1,600 calories	1,700 calories
	LUNCH				
Corned Beef (3 ounces extra-lean) on 2 slices rye bread with favorite mustard	Use 1 slice rye bread	Use 1 slice rye bread	1 serving	1 serving	1 serving
Mixed green salad with Italian dressing (1 cup romaine lettuce, $1/2$ cup chopped tomatoes, $1/2$ cup chopped onions, 2 tablespoons Italian dressing)	1 serving	1 serving	1 serving	1 serving	1 serving
Coffee	As desired	As desired	As desired	As desired	As desired
	AFTERNOON SNACK				
Fresh apricots	1	1	2	2	2
	DINNER				
Chicken-Veggie Stir-Fry over Linguine	$1/2$ recipe	$1/2$ recipe	$1/2$ recipe	$1/2$ recipe	$1/2$ recipe
Skim milk	$1/2$ cup	$1/2$ cup	$1/2$ cup	$1/2$ cup	$1/2$ cup
Raspberry Cheesecake	1 slice	1 slice	1 slice	1 slice	1 slice
	EVENING SNACK				
Apple	Omit	1	1	1	1
	NUTRITION TOTALS FOR DAY SEVEN				
Calories	1,279	1,360	1,503	1,629	1,679
Fat (g)	42	43	44	47	53
Carbohydrates (g)	144	165	190	213	213
Protein (g)	89	90	97	99	99
Fiber (g)	15	19	22	23	24
Cals. from fat (%)	29	27	26	25	28

	WEEK THREE				
	Week Three, Day One				
Food	1,300 calories	1,400 calories	1,500 calories	1,600 calories	1,700 calories
BREAKFAST					
Poached egg	1	1	1	1	1
Whole wheat English muffin	1	1	1	1	1
Light tub margarine	2 teaspoons	1 tablespoon	1 tablespoon	1 tablespoon	1 tablespoon
Hot herbal tea	As desired	As desired	As desired	As desired	As desired
MORNING SNACK					
Cafe mocha: 1/2 cup skim milk, heated; 1 tablespoon unsweetened cocoa powder; 1 packet artificial sweetener; 1/2 cup strong hot coffee	1 serving	1 serving	1 serving	Use 1 cup skim milk; 2 tablespoons unsweetened cocoa powder; 2 packets artificial sweetener; and 1 cup strong hot coffee	1 cup skim milk; 2 tablespoons unsweetened cocoa powder; 2 packets artificial sweetener; and 1 cup strong hot coffee
LUNCH					
Whole wheat bagel	1/2	1/2	1	1	1
Peanut butter	2 tablespoons	2 tablespoons	2 tablespoons	2 tablespoons	2 tablespoons
Skim milk	1/2 cup	1/2 cup	1 cup	1 cup	1 cup
AFTERNOON SNACK					
Favorite flavored seltzer water	As desired	As desired	As desired	As desired	As desired
Apple	1	1	1	1	1
DINNER					
Parsnip Whipped Potatoes	1/8 recipe	1/8 recipe	1/8 recipe	1/8 recipe	1/8 recipe
Grilled Asparagus and Leeks	1/6 recipe	1/6 recipe	1/6 recipe	1/6 recipe	1/6 recipe
Broiled tenderloin	3 ounces	3 ounces	3 ounces	3 ounces	3 ounces

Food	1,300 calories	1,400 calories	1,500 calories	1,600 calories	1,700 calories
Peach Creamsicle Sundae with Marion Blackberry Fruit Perfect	¹/₄ recipe	¹/₄ recipe	¹/₄ recipe	¹/₄ recipe	¹/₄ recipe
Perrier with fresh lime	As desired	As desired	As desired	As desired	As desired

EVENING SNACK

	1,300 calories	1,400 calories	1,500 calories	1,600 calories	1,700 calories
Cantaloupe	¹/₄ melon	¹/₄ melon	¹/₄ melon	¹/₄ melon	¹/₄ melon
Fat-free vanilla yogurt	Omit	¹/₄ cup	¹/₄ cup	¹/₂ cup	1 cup

NUTRITION TOTALS FOR DAY ONE

	1,300 calories	1,400 calories	1,500 calories	1,600 calories	1,700 calories
Calories	1,297	1,366	1,481	1,588	1,692
Fat (g)	45	48	48	50	50
Carbohydrates (g)	170	180	202	221	242
Protein (g)	70	73	80	88	93
Fiber (g)	26	27	29	32	33
Cals. from fat (%)	30	30	28	27	25

Week Three, Day Two

Food	1,300 calories	1,400 calories	1,500 calories	1,600 calories	1,700 calories

BREAKFAST

Food	1,300 calories	1,400 calories	1,500 calories	1,600 calories	1,700 calories
Favorite flavor instant oatmeal (prepare with milk instead of water for extra creaminess)	1 packet	1 packet	1 packet	1 packet	1 packet
Skim milk	1 cup	1 cup	1 cup	1 cup	1 cup
Slivered almonds	2 tablespoons	3 tablespoons	3 tablespoons	3 tablespoons	3 tablespoons

MORNING SNACK

	1,300 calories	1,400 calories	1,500 calories	1,600 calories	1,700 calories
Large fresh orange	1	1	1	1	1

			Week Three, Day Two (continued)		
Food	1,300 calories	1,400 calories	1,500 calories	1,600 calories	1,700 calories
LUNCH					
Canned lentil pasta soup	2 cups	2 cups	2 cups	2 cups	2 cups
Whole wheat pita, toasted	$^1/_2$	I	I	I	I
Light tub margarine	I tablespoon	I tablespoon	I tablespoon	I tablespoon	I tablespoon
Iced seltzer water	As desired	As desired	As desired	As desired	As desired
AFTERNOON SNACK					
Banana	Omit	Omit	$^1/_2$	$^1/_2$	I
DINNER					
Shrimp Slaw with Jicama, Pineapple, and Watercress	$^1/_6$ recipe	$^1/_6$ recipe	$^1/_6$ recipe	$^1/_6$ recipe	$^1/_6$ recipe
Herb-Seared Day Boat Cod with Fresh Stewed Tomatoes	$^1/_6$ recipe	$^1/_6$ recipe	$^1/_6$ recipe	$^1/_6$ recipe	$^1/_6$ recipe
Linguine	$^1/_2$ cup	$^1/_2$ cup	$^1/_2$ cup	$^1/_2$ cup	$^3/_4$ cup
Butter	Omit	Omit	I teaspoon for linguine	I tablespoon for linguine	I tablespoon for linguine
Warm Pear and Blueberry Granola Crisp with Maple Yogurt	$^1/_6$ recipe	$^1/_6$ recipe	$^1/_6$ recipe	$^1/_6$ recipe	$^1/_6$ recipe
EVENING SNACK					
Hot herbal tea	As desired	As desired	As desired	As desired	As desired
NUTRITION TOTALS FOR DAY TWO					
Calories	1,318	1,401	1,554	1,622	1,721
Fat (g)	31	32	39	46	47
Carbohydrates (g)	190	208	229	229	252
Protein (g)	73	77	78	78	81
Fiber (g)	27	28	33	33	35
Cals from fat (%)	21	20	22	26	24

Week Three, Day Three

1,300 Food	1,400 calories	1,500 calories	1,600 calories	1,700 calories	calories
BREAKFAST					
High-fiber cereal	¹/₂ cup	¹/₂ cup	¹/₂ cup	¹/₂ cup	¹/₂ cup
Dried cranberries	2 tablespoons	2 tablespoons	2 tablespoons	2 tablespoons	2 tablespoons
Chopped walnuts	2 tablespoons	3 tablespoons	3 tablespoons	4 tablespoons	4 tablespoons
Skim milk	¹/₂ cup	¹/₂ cup	¹/₂ cup	¹/₂ cup	¹/₂ cup
MORNING SNACK					
Large fresh peach	I	I	I	I	I
LUNCH					
Pita Stuffed with Peanut Butter and Banana	Recipe as shown	Recipe as shown	Recipe as shown	Recipe as shown	Use whole pita pocket
Vegetable juice cocktail	Omit	12 ounces	12 ounces	12 ounces	12 ounces
AFTERNOON SNACK					
Hot herbal tea	As desired	As desired	As desired	As desired	As desired
Skim milk	I cup	I cup	I cup	I cup	I cup
Fresh apricots	Omit	2	2	2	2
DINNER					
Breast of Chicken with Braised White Beans and Arugula	¹/₄ recipe	¹/₄ recipe	¹/₄ recipe	¹/₄ recipe	¹/₄ recipe
Whole wheat dinner roll	I	I	I	I	I
Butter	I teaspoon	I teaspoon	I teaspoon	I teaspoon	2 teaspoons
EVENING SNACK					
Decaffeinated coffee with pure vanilla extract and artificial sweetener	As desired	As desired	As desired	As desired	As desired
Raisin Nut Bran cereal	Omit	Omit	¹/₃ cup	¹/₂ cup	¹/₂ cup
Skim milk	Omit	Omit	¹/₃ cup	¹/₃ cup	¹/₂ cup

Week Three, Day Three (continued)

NUTRITION TOTALS FOR DAY THREE

Calories	1,277	1,422	1,521	1,604	1,738
Fat (g)	43	48	50	56	60
Carbohydrates (g)	152	176	193	201	220
Protein (g)	83	88	93	95	100
Fiber (g)	31	36	38	39	41
Cals. from fat (%)	29	29	28	30	30

Week Three, Day Four

Food	1,300 calories	1,400 calories	1,500 calories	1,600 calories	1,700 calories
			BREAKFAST		
12-grain toast	1	1	1	1	1
Cashew butter	2 tablespoons	2 tablespoons	2 tablespoons	2 tablespoons	2 tablespoons
Favorite marmalade	1 tablespoon	1 tablespoon	1 tablespoon	1 tablespoon	1 tablespoon
Coffee	As desired	As desired	As desired	As desired	As desired
			MORNING SNACK		
Hot chocolate (made with skim milk, 1 tablespoon unsweetened cocoa, 1 packet artificial sweetener, and vanilla extract to taste)	½ cup	½ cup	½ cup	½ cup	½ cup
			LUNCH		
Frozen reduced-fat French bread pizza (such as Lean Cuisine)	1 serving	1 serving	1 serving	1 serving	1 serving
Spinach salad (made with 2 cups baby spinach leaves and 10 cherry tomatoes)	Serve with 2 tablespoons low-fat Italian dressing	Serve with 1½ tablespoons regular Italian dressing	Serve with 1½ tablespoons regular Italian dressing	Serve with 1½ tablespoons regular Italian dressing	Serve with 2 tablespoons regular Italian dressing
Iced seltzer water	As desired	As desired	As desired	As desired	As desired

Food	1,300 calories	1,400 calories	1,500 calories	1,600 calories	1,700 calories
AFTERNOON SNACK					
Nonfat fruited yogurt (100 calories per 8-ounce serving)	Omit	Omit	8 ounces	8 ounces	8 ounces
DINNER					
Penne with Grilled Chicken and Forest Mushrooms	⅙ recipe	⅙ recipe	⅙ recipe	⅙ recipe	⅙ recipe
Old-Fashioned Apple and Fresh Raspberry Cobbler	⅛ recipe	⅛ recipe	⅛ recipe	⅛ recipe	⅛ recipe
Hot tea	As desired	As desired	As desired	As desired	As desired
EVENING SNACK					
Oat bran pretzels	Omit	Omit	Omit	1 ounce	1 ounce
Orange juice spritzer (½ cup orange juice plus ½ cup plain iced seltzer water)	Omit	Omit	Omit	Omit	1 serving
NUTRITION TOTALS FOR DAY FOUR					
Calories	1,370	1,441	1,535	1,648	1,745
Fat (g)	35	43	44	46	49
Carbohydrates (g)	204	204	219	241	255
Protein (g)	71	71	81	83	83
Fiber (g)	23	23	23	25	25
Cals. from fat (%)	22	26	25	24	25

Week Three, Day Five

Food	1,300 calories	1,400 calories	1,500 calories	1,600 calories	1,700 calories
BREAKFAST					
Cheese Tomato Omelet	Recipe as shown	Recipe as shown	Recipe as shown	Recipe as shown	Recipe as shown
12-grain toast	2 slices	2 slices	2 slices	2 slices	2 slices
Favorite jam	1 tablespoon	1 tablespoon	1 tablespoon	1 tablespoon	1 tablespoon

Food	1,300 calories	1,400 calories	1,500 calories	1,600 calories	1,700 calories
Week Three, Day Five (continued)					
MORNING SNACK					
Hot herbal tea	As desired	As desired	As desired	As desired	As desired
Fresh papaya with freshly squeezed lemon juice	Omit	Omit	Omit	Omit	1
LUNCH					
Kris's Split Pea Soup	1/8 recipe	1/8 recipe	1/8 recipe	1/8 recipe	1/8 recipe
Pita bread	Omit	Omit	1/2	1/2	1/2
Peanut butter	Omit	Omit	1 teaspoon	1 tablespoon	1 tablespoon
AFTERNOON SNACK					
Nonfat fruited yogurt (100 cals. per 8 ounces)	8 ounces	8 ounces	8 ounces	8 ounces	8 ounces
DINNER					
Frozen veggie burger	1	1	1	1	1
Whole wheat bun	1	1	1	1	1
Blue cheese salad dressing	1 tablespoon	2 tablespoons	2 tablespoons	2 tablespoons	2 tablespoons
Tomato and red onion slices	As desired	As desired	As desired	As desired	As desired
EVENING SNACK					
Sliced strawberries	Omit	1 cup	1 cup	1 cup	1 cup
NUTRITION TOTALS FOR DAY FIVE					
Calories	1,310	1,437	1,554	1,616	1,735
Fat (g)	33	42	45	51	51
Carbohydrates (g)	176	189	238	210	240
Protein (g)	83	84	89	91	93
Fiber (g)	15	19	27	22	27
Cals. from fat (%)	22	26	26	27	26

Food	*1,300 calories*	*1,400 calories*	*1,500 calories*	*1,600 calories*	*1,700 calories*
		Week Three, Day Six			
BREAKFAST					
Pita Stuffed with Egg, Cheese, and Bacon	Recipe as shown	Recipe as shown	Recipe as shown	Recipe as shown	Recipe as shown
Orange juice	8 ounces	8 ounces	8 ounces	8 ounces	8 ounces
MORNING SNACK					
Apple	1	1	1	1	1
Fat-free cream cheese	Omit	Omit	Omit	1 tablespoon (placed on sliced apple and embedded with dried cranberries)	1 tablespoon (placed on sliced apple and embedded with dried cranberries)
Dried cranberries	Omit	Omit	Omit	1 tablespoon	1 tablespoon
LUNCH					
Grilled Ham and Cheese	Recipe as shown	Recipe as shown	Recipe as shown	Recipe as shown	Recipe as shown
Skim milk	Omit	1 cup	1 cup	1 cup	1 cup
Sweet red pepper, sliced	1	1	1	1	1
Peppercorn ranch dressing for dipping sweet red pepper	2 tablespoons	2 tablespoons	2 tablespoons	2 tablespoons	2 tablespoons
AFTERNOON SNACK					
Favorite iced coffee	As desired	As desired	As desired	As desired	As desired

Week Three, Day Six (continued)

Food	1,300 calories	1,400 calories	1,500 calories	1,600 calories	1,700 calories
DINNER					
Barbecued chicken (3 ounces with 2 tablespoons sauce)	I serving	I serving	I serving	I serving	I serving
Corn on the cob	I	I	I	I	I
Butter for corn	2 teaspoons	I tablespoon	I tablespoon	I tablespoon	I tablespoon
Mixed green salad (2 cups lettuce, ½ cup chopped tomatoes, ½ cup chopped onions, 2 tablespoons Italian dressing)	I serving	I serving	I serving	I serving	I serving
EVENING SNACK					
Fresh blueberries	½ cup	½ cup	½ cup	½ cup	½ cup
Sliced strawberries	Omit	Omit	I cup	I cup	I cup
Low-fat lemon yogurt for topping	Omit	Omit	¼ cup	½ cup	I cup
NUTRITION TOTALS FOR DAY SIX					
Calories	1,302	1,426	1,528	1,618	1,723
Fat (g)	36	41	42	43	44
Carbohydrates (g)	170	182	202	217	234
Protein (g)	83	92	96	101	107
Fiber (g)	24	24	28	28	28
Cals. from fat (%)	24	25	24	23	23

Week Three, Day Seven

Food	1,300 calories	1,400 calories	1,500 calories	1,600 calories	1,700 calories
BREAKFAST					
Fiber One cereal	½ cup	½ cup	½ cup	½ cup	½ cup
Dried cranberries	2 tablespoons	2 tablespoons	2 tablespoons	2 tablespoons	2 tablespoons
Chopped walnuts	2 tablespoon	2 tablespoons	2 tablespoons	2 tablespoons	2 tablespoons
Skim milk	I cup	I cup	I cup	I cup	I cup

Food	1,300 calories	1,400 calories	1,500 calories	1,600 calories	1,700 calories
			MORNING SNACK		
Hot herbal tea	As desired	As desired	As desired	As desired	As desired
Oat bran pretzels	Omit	Omit	Omit	1 ounce	1 ounce
			LUNCH		
Spicy Bean Tortilla	Recipe as shown	Recipe as shown	Recipe as shown	Recipe as shown	Recipe as shown
Low-fat coffee yogurt	1/2 cup	1 cup	1 cup	1 cup	1 cup
			AFTERNOON SNACK		
Baby carrots	10	10	10	10	10
Favorite low-fat salad dressing for dipping	2 tablespoons	2 tablespoons	2 tablespoons	2 tablespoons	2 tablespoons
			DINNER		
Frozen chicken enchilada dinner (such as Lean Cuisine)	1	1	1	1	1
Frozen corn	1 cup	1 cup	1 cup	1 cup	1 cup
Butter for corn	Omit	Omit	Omit	Omit	2 teaspoons
			EVENING SNACK		
Fresh or frozen raspberries	Omit	1 cup	1 cup	1 cup	1 cup
Low-fat vanilla yogurt for raspberries	Omit	1/4 cup	1/4 cup	1/4 cup	2 teaspoons
			NUTRITION TOTALS FOR DAY SEVEN		
Calories	1,332	1,437	1,550	1,663	1,731
Fat (g)	38	40	41	42	50
Carbohydrates (g)	203	220	243	265	265
Protein (g)	60	66	70	73	73
Fiber (g)	35	35	43	45	45
Cals. from fat (%)	24	24	23	22	25

	WEEK FOUR				
	Week Four, Day One				
Food	*1,300* calories	*1,400* calories	*1,500* calories	*1,600* calories	*1,700* calories
BREAKFAST					
Slivered almonds	2 tablespoons	2 tablespoons	3 tablespoons	3 tablespoons	3 tablespoons
Raisins	2 tablespoons	2 tablespoons	3 tablespoons	3 tablespoons	3 tablespoons
Low-fat yogurt	I cup	I cup	I cup	I cup	I cup
MORNING SNACK					
Fresh orange	I	I	I	I	I
LUNCH					
Frozen veggie burger on whole wheat bun	I	I	I	I	I
Garnish for veggie burger: at least 2 slices tomato, 2 leaves romaine lettuce, mustard as desired	As indicated	As indicated	As indicated	As indicated	As indicated
Iced tea	As desired	As desired	As desired	As desired	As desired
AFTERNOON SNACK					
Banana	I	I	I	I	I
DINNER					
Grilled tuna steak	3 ounces	3 ounces	3 ounces	4 ounces	5 ounces
Baked sweet potato	I	I	I	I	I
Butter for sweet potato	I teaspoon	I tablespoon	I tablespoon	I tablespoon	I tablespoon
Brown sugar for sweet potato	Omit	Omit	Omit	I tablespoon	I tablespoon
Asparagus spears	6	6	6	6	6
Hot tea	As desired	As desired	As desired	As desired	As desired
EVENING SNACK					
Fresh or frozen raspberries	Omit	$^1/_2$ cup	$^3/_4$ cup	$^3/_4$ cup	I cup
Skim milk	I cup	I cup	I cup	I cup	I cup

NUTRITION TOTALS FOR DAY ONE

Calories	1,301	1,399	1,497	1,601	1,699
Fat (g)	30	38	42	44	46
Carbohydrates (g)	192	200	213	226	238
Protein (g)	75	76	78	86	95
Fiber (g)	25	29	32	32	35
Cals. from fat (%)	20	24	25	24	24

Week Four, Day Two

Food	1,300 calories	1,400 calories	1,500 calories	1,600 calories	1,700 calories
BREAKFAST					
Pita Stuffed with Egg, Cheese, and Bacon	1	1	1	1	1
Coffee	As desired	As desired	As desired	As desired	As desired
MORNING SNACK					
Herbal tea	As desired	As desired	As desired	As desired	As desired
LUNCH					
Peanut Butter and Banana Breakfast Smoothie	Recipe as shown	Recipe as shown	Recipe as shown	Recipe as shown	Recipe as shown
Fruit salad: 1 cup strawberries and 1 sliced kiwi	As indicated	As indicated	As indicated	As indicated	As indicated
AFTERNOON SNACK					
Apple	1	1	1	1	1
DINNER					
Roast beef, lean	3 ounces	3 ounces	4 ounces	4 ounces	4 ounces
Sour Cream and Chives Baked Potato	1	1	1	1	1
Romaine lettuce with 1 tablespoon balsamic vinegar and freshly ground black pepper	As desired	As desired	As desired	As desired	As desired

Week Four, Day Two (continued)				
Food	1,300 calories	1,400 calories	1,500 calories	1,600 calories	1,700 calories
DINNER					
Green peas	Omit	Omit	Omit	I cup	I cup
Butter for peas	Omit	Omit	Omit	Omit	I teaspoon
Hot tea	As desired	As desired	As desired	As desired	As desired
EVENING SNACK					
Nonfat fruited yogurt (100 calories per 8 ounces)	Omit	8 ounces	8 ounces	8 ounces	8 ounces
NUTRITION TOTALS FOR DAY TWO					
Calories	1,380	1,473	1,523	1,647	1,681
Fat (g)	42	42	44	44	48
Carbohydrates (g)	180	194	194	217	217
Protein (g)	87	96	105	113	113
Fiber (g)	27	27	27	36	36
Cals. from fat (%)	26	25	25	23	25

Week Four, Day Three				
Food	1,300 calories	1,400 calories	1,500 calories	1,600 calories	1,700 calories
BREAKFAST					
Poached egg	I	I	I	I	I
Whole wheat bagel	I	I	I	I	I
Light tub margarine	I teaspoon	2 teaspoons	2 teaspoons	2 teaspoons	2 teaspoons
MORNING SNACK					
Hot chocolate: (made with I cup skim milk, 2 tablespoons unsweetened cocoa, and I packet artificial sweetener)	I serving	I serving	I serving	I serving	I serving

Food	1,300 calories	1,400 calories	1,500 calories	1,600 calories	1,700 calories
LUNCH					
Kris's Split Pea Soup	I serving	I serving	I serving	I serving	I serving
Soy nuts	¼ cup	¼ cup	¼ cup	¼ cup	¼ cup
Coffee	As desired	As desired	As desired	As desired	As desired
AFTERNOON SNACK					
Fresh peach	I	I	I	I	I
DINNER					
Herb-Seared Day Boat Cod with Fresh Stewed Tomatoes	I serving	I serving	I serving	I serving	I serving
Brown rice	½ cup	½ cup	½ cup	½ cup	I cup
Steamed broccoli with lemon juice	I cup	I cup	I cup	I cup	I cup
EVENING SNACK					
Kiwi	I	I	I	I	I
Low-fat vanilla yogurt	Omit	Omit	½ cup	I cup	I cup
NUTRITION TOTALS FOR DAY THREE					
Calories	1,312	1,422	1,527	1,632	1,740
Fat (g)	21	25	26	28	29
Carbohydrates (g)	187	199	215	232	255
Protein (g)	101	110	116	122	124
Fiber (g)	19	19	19	19	20
Cals. from fat (%)	14	15	15	15	15

Week Four, Day Four					
Food	1,300 calories	1,400 calories	1,500 calories	1,600 calories	1,700 calories
BREAKFAST					
Strawberry-Banana-Kiwi Smoothie	Recipe as shown	Recipe as shown	Recipe as shown	Recipe as shown	Recipe as shown
Cinnamon raisin bagel	Omit	½	I	I	I

Week Four, Day Four (continued)

Food	1,300 calories	1,400 calories	1,500 calories	1,600 calories	1,700 calories
MORNING SNACK					
Plums	2	2	2	2	2
LUNCH					
Peanut butter and jelly sandwich: 2 slices whole wheat bread, 2 tablespoons peanut butter, and 1 tablespoon jelly	As indicated	As indicated	As indicated	As indicated	As indicated
Skim milk	Omit	Omit	Omit	Omit	1 cup
Baby carrots and celery sticks	As desired	As desired	As desired	As desired	As desired
AFTERNOON SNACK					
Banana	1	1	1	1	1
DINNER					
Grilled salmon with fresh lime juice	3 ounces	3 ounces	4 ounces	4 ounces	4 ounces
Steamed cauliflower with lemon juice and freshly chopped parsley	1 cup	1 cup	1 cup	1 cup	1 cup
Sweet potato	1	1	1	1	1
Butter for sweet potato	2 teaspoons	2 teaspoons	2 teaspoons	2 teaspoons	2 teaspoons
EVENING SNACK					
Herbal tea	As desired	As desired	As desired	As desired	As desired
Fat-free Fig Newton	Omit	Omit	Omit	1	1
NUTRITION TOTALS FOR DAY FOUR					
Calories	1,298	1,395	1,554	1,622	1,707
Fat (g)	42	43	46	46	47
Carbohydrates (g)	192	212	232	247	259
Protein (g)	56	60	71	72	80
Fiber (g)	28	29	30	30	30
Cals. from fat (%)	28	26	26	25	24

Week Four, Day Five

Food	1,300 calories	1,400 calories	1,500 calories	1,600 calories	1,700 calories
BREAKFAST					
Cinnamon raisin English muffin	1	1	1	1	1
Butter	2 teaspoons	1 tablespoon	1 tablespoon	1 tablespoon	1 tablespoon
¹/₂ grapefruit with 1 teaspoon sugar	Omit	Omit	As indicated	As indicated	As indicated
MORNING SNACK					
Fresh apricots	2	2	2	2	2
LUNCH					
Frozen honey mustard chicken (such as Lean Cuisine)	1	1	1	1	1
Spinach salad: 2 cups spinach, whole tomato (chopped), 2 tablespoons favorite regular dressing	As indicated	As indicated	As indicated	As indicated	As indicated
AFTERNOON SNACK					
Orange	1	1	1	1	1
DINNER					
Lemon, Basil, and Ginger Tofu Stir-Fry with Spinach Rotini	1 serving	1 serving	1 serving	1 serving	1 serving
Italian bread	Omit	Omit	Omit	1-ounce slice	1-ounce slice
Butter for bread	Omit	Omit	Omit	1 teaspoon	1 teaspoon
EVENING SNACK					
Fresh raspberries	¹/₂ cup	¹/₂ cup	¹/₂ cup	¹/₂ cup	¹/₂ cup
Fat-free chocolate sorbet	Omit	Omit	Omit	Omit	¹/₂ cup
NUTRITION TOTALS FOR DAY FIVE					
Calories	1,286	1,437	1,492	1,603	1,713
Fat (g)	45	49	49	54	54
Carbohydrates (g)	179	200	214	228	256
Protein (g)	59	66	67	70	71
Fiber (g)	27	35	36	37	39
Cals. from fat (%)	30	29	28	29	27

Week Four, Day Six					
Food	1,300 calories	1,400 calories	1,500 calories	1,600 calories	1,700 calories
BREAKFAST					
Raisin Bran cereal	1 cup	1 cup	1 cup	1 cup	1 cup
Slivered almonds for cereal	2 tablespoons	2 tablespoons	2 tablespoons	2 tablespoons	2 tablespoons
Skim milk	1 cup	1 cup	1 cup	1 cup	1 cup
MORNING SNACK					
Seltzer water	As desired	As desired	As desired	As desired	As desired
LUNCH					
Low-fat frozen French bread pizza (such as Lean Cuisine)	1 slice	1 slice	1 slice	1 slice	1 slice
Trail mix: 2 tablespoons peanuts, 2 tablespoons raisins, 1 tablespoon chocolate chips	As indicated	As indicated	As indicated	As indicated	As indicated
AFTERNOON SNACK					
Hot tea	As desired	As desired	As desired	As desired	As desired
Grapes	Omit	1 cup	1 cup	1 cup	1 cup
DINNER					
Grilled beef tenderloin	3 ounces	3 ounces	3 ounces	3 ounces	3 ounces
Baked potato	1	1	1	1	1
Butter for potato	2 teaspoons	2 teaspoons	2 teaspoons	2 teaspoons	2 teaspoons
Steamed carrot slices with fresh parsley	1 cup	1 cup	1 cup	1 cup	1 cup
Skim milk	Omit	Omit	Omit	1 cup	1 cup

Food	1,300 calories	1,400 calories	1,500 calories	1,600 calories	1,700 calories
			EVENING SNACK		
Fruit sorbet	Omit	Omit	Omit	Omit	½ cup
Apple	Omit	1	1	1	1

NUTRITION TOTALS FOR DAY SIX

	1,300 calories	1,400 calories	1,500 calories	1,600 calories	1,700 calories
Calories	1,328	1,357	1,471	1,608	1,700
Fat (g)	46	42	43	48	48
Carbohydrates (g)	171	191	219	233	256
Protein (g)	71	69	70	81	81
Fiber (g)	22	25	27	28	28
Cals. from fat (%)	30	27	25	25	24

Week Four, Day Seven

Food	1,300 calories	1,400 calories	1,500 calories	1,600 calories	1,700 calories
			BREAKFAST		
Cheese omelet (made with 1 egg and 1 ounce 50% reduced-fat cheese)	1 serving	1 serving	Use 2 eggs	Use 2 eggs	Use 2 eggs
Whole wheat toast	1 slice	2 slices	2 slices	2 slices	2 slices
Light tub margarine	1 teaspoon	2 teaspoons	2 teaspoons	2 teaspoons	2 teaspoons
			MORNING SNACK		
Grapes	1 cup	1 cup	1 cup	1 cup	1 cup
			LUNCH		
Turkey sandwich: 2 slices rye bread, 3 ounces turkey breast, romaine lettuce, 2 tablespoons low-fat mayonnaise	As indicated	As indicated	As indicated	As indicated	As indicated
Skim milk	1 cup	1 cup	1 cup	1 cup	1 cup

Food	1,300 calories	1,400 calories	1,500 calories	1,600 calories	1,700 calories
Week Four, Day Seven (continued)					
AFTERNOON SNACK					
Plums	1	1	2	2	2
DINNER					
Chicken Stir-Fry	Recipe as shown	Recipe as shown	Recipe as shown	Recipe as shown	Recipe as shown
Brown rice	½ cup	½ cup	½ cup	½ cup	½ cup
Broccoli with 1 teaspoon butter and freshly chopped chives	1 cup	1 cup	1 cup	1 cup	1 cup
Skim milk	Omit	Omit	Omit	Omit	1 cup
EVENING SNACK					
Strawberries	Omit	Omit	Omit	1 cup	1 cup
Low-fat whipped topping	Omit	Omit	Omit	2 tablespoons	2 tablespoons
NUTRITION TOTALS FOR DAY SEVEN					
Calories	1,338	1,432	1,543	1,613	1,698
Fat (g)	40	44	49	51	51
Carbohydrates (g)	156	169	178	192	204
Protein (g)	101	103	110	111	119
Fiber (g)	23	26	27	30	30
Cals. from fat (%)	26	26	28	27	26

Recipes

Before preparing our delicious, nutritious recipes, please take the time to note these three points:

1. Although you probably don't need a recipe to prepare a roast beef sandwich or a mixed salad, you will find such recipes here because paying close attention to portion sizes is key to your success when following our diet plan.

2. Depending on the calorie level you have chosen to follow, you may need to change the amounts of certain ingredients slightly. This is

noted in the menu plans, and those ingredients are denoted in the recipes by an asterisk.

3. All recipes are organized in the categories and in the order that they appear in our menus. Special desserts follow the dinner recipes.

FOR BREAKFAST

Strawberry-Banana-Kiwi Breakfast Smoothie

SERVES 1

$\frac{1}{2}$ cup low-fat yogurt
1 banana, cut into chunks
1 cup frozen strawberries (not thawed)
2 tablespoons wheat germ
1 kiwi, peeled and cut into chunks

Place all the ingredients in a blender and blend until smooth.

Per serving: 338 calories, 4.5 grams fat, 68 grams carbohydrate, 13 grams protein, 10 grams fiber.

Peanut Butter and Banana Breakfast Smoothie

SERVES 1

$\frac{1}{2}$ cup low-fat vanilla yogurt
1 tablespoon peanut butter
$\frac{1}{2}$ banana, cut into chunks
1 tablespoon wheat germ

Place all the ingredients in a blender and blend until smooth.

VARIATION: Use $\frac{3}{4}$ cup low-fat soy milk instead of yogurt with 1 tablespoon peanut butter and 1 banana. Omit wheat germ.

Per serving: 420 calories, 18 grams fat, 47 grams carbohydrate, 18 grams protein, 6 grams fiber

Oatmeal with Apple and Brown Sugar

SERVES I

1/2 cup old-fashioned or quick-cooking oats
I cup skim milk
I apple (with peel), chopped
I teaspoon packed brown sugar
I tablespoon wheat germ

Combine the oats, milk, and apple, and cook according to the package directions. Top with the brown sugar and wheat germ.

Per serving: 366 calories, 4 grams fat, 68 grams carbohydrate, 17 grams protein, 9 grams fiber

Western Omelet

SERVES I

I egg plus 2 egg whites
1/2 cup sliced mushrooms
1/4 cup chopped green onion
1/4 cup chopped tomato

Combine all the ingredients and cook in a nonstick pan coated with vegetable oil spray until desired dryness is reached.

Per serving: 125 calories, 5 grams fat, 7 grams carbohydrate, 14 grams protein, 2 grams fiber,

Raspberry-Vanilla Smoothie

SERVES I

1/2 cup low-fat vanilla yogurt
I cup frozen unsweetened raspberries*

Place the ingredients in a blender and blend until smooth.

Per serving: 207 calories, 2 grams fat, 40 grams carbohydrate, 10 grams protein, 12 grams fiber

Green Pepper Omelet

SERVES 1

2 eggs*
1 green bell pepper, minced
ground black pepper to taste

Coat a nonstick pan with vegetable oil spray and heat over medium heat. Beat the eggs slightly and pour into the pan. Just when the eggs start to congeal, add the green pepper. Cover and cook 5 minutes, or until the eggs are entirely cooked. Add pepper, remove the omelet from the pan, and fold in half. Season to taste with black pepper.

Per serving: 169 calories, 10 grams fat, 6 grams carbohydrate, 13 grams protein, 1 gram fiber

Banana Almond Oatmeal

SERVES 1

1/2 cup old-fashioned or quick-cooking oats
1 cup skim milk
1 banana, sliced
2 tablespoons slivered almonds*

Combine the oats and milk. Cook according to the directions on the oatmeal container. Top with the banana slices and almonds.

Per serving: 453 calories, 12 grams fat, 69 grams carbohydrate, 19 grams protein, 9 grams fiber

Breakfast Peanut Fruit Salad

SERVES 1

1 banana, sliced*
1 kiwi, peeled and sliced
1 cup low-fat vanilla yogurt*
2 tablespoons chopped peanuts*

Combine the fruit and toss with the yogurt. Sprinkle with the chopped peanuts.

Per serving: 460 calories, 12 grams fat, 75 grams carbohydrate, 18 grams protein, 7 grams fiber

The Moistest Pumpkin Muffins

MAKES 3 DOZEN MUFFINS, OR 2 LARGE LOAVES

Stores well in the freezer up to three months.

$\frac{1}{3}$ cup applesauce
$\frac{1}{3}$ cup canola or olive oil
$2\frac{2}{3}$ cups sugar
4 eggs (or the equivalent in egg substitute)
I can (16 ounces) pumpkin
$\frac{2}{3}$ cup nonfat plain yogurt
$\frac{2}{3}$ cup wheat germ
$1\frac{2}{3}$ cups whole wheat flour
I cup white flour
2 teaspoons baking soda
$\frac{1}{2}$ teaspoon baking powder
I teaspoon ground cinnamon
I teaspoon ground cloves
$\frac{1}{2}$ cup milled flaxseed

Combine the applesauce, oil, sugar, eggs, pumpkin, yogurt, and wheat germ in a large mixing bowl. Mix on medium speed until well blended. Add the remaining ingredients and mix just until the flour is blended in.

Fill 36 muffin tins $\frac{2}{3}$ full or divide the batter between 2 large loaf pans.

Bake at 350 degrees for about 20–30 minutes for muffins or 70 minutes for loaves, until a knife inserted in the middle comes out clean.

Per serving (1 muffin): 132 calories, 3 grams fat, 24 grams carbohydrate, 3 grams protein, 2 grams fiber

Cheese Tomato Omelet

SERVES 1

1 egg, slightly beaten
1 ounce sharp cheddar cheese
$\frac{1}{2}$ tomato, chopped

Heat a nonstick pan coated with vegetable oil spray over medium heat. Add the beaten egg.

Just when the egg starts to congeal, add the cheese and tomato. Do not cover. Allow the egg to cook and the cheese to melt.

Per serving: 201 calories, 15 grams fat, 4 grams carbohydrate, 14 grams protein, 1 gram fiber

Pita Stuffed with Egg, Cheese, and Bacon

SERVES 1

1 egg, poached
1 slice reduced-fat American cheese
1 ounce lean Canadian bacon, cooked in a microwave
1 whole pita pocket with top sliced off and toasted

Place the egg, cheese, and bacon in the pita pocket and serve.

Per serving: 348 calories, 11 grams fat, 37 grams carbohydrate, 26 grams protein, 5 grams fiber

FOR LUNCH

Tuna Fish on Pita

SERVES 1

2 ounces tuna packed in water
2 tablespoons light mayonnaise
$\frac{1}{2}$ whole wheat pita pocket
1 cup chopped romaine lettuce leaves
$\frac{1}{2}$ cup chopped tomato

Flake the tuna and use a fork to combine it with the mayonnaise. Stuff the mixture in a pita pocket with the lettuce and tomato.

Per serving: 245 calories, 7 grams fat, 28 grams carbohydrate, 19 grams protein, 4 grams fiber

Fresh Garden Salad with Balsamic Vinaigrette

SERVES 1

Salad:
2 cups chopped romaine lettuce
1/2 tomato, chopped
1/2 cup canned garbanzo beans, drained*
1 carrot, grated
1/2 sweet green pepper, chopped
1/4 cup chopped green onions

Dressing:
2 tablespoons balsamic vinegar
1 tablespoon extra-virgin olive oil
1 teaspoon sugar
freshly ground black pepper to taste
1/4 cup chopped fresh cilantro or basil

Toss all the salad ingredients together. Combine the dressing ingredients and pour over the salad.

Per serving: 370 calories, 17 grams fat, 48 grams carbohydrate, 9 grams protein, 13 grams fiber

Lean Turkey Sandwich on Whole Wheat

SERVES 1

2 ounces lean turkey breast
1 cup fresh spinach leaves
2 slices whole wheat bread*
1 tablespoon light mayonnaise

Assemble the sandwich with the ingredients.

Per serving: 275 calories, 6 grams fat, 33 grams carbohydrate, 24 grams protein, 5 grams fiber

Spicy Bean Tortilla

SERVES 1

1 large flour tortilla*
1/2 cup canned fat-free refried beans
1 ounce taco cheese
1/2 green pepper, chopped
1/2 cup tomato, chopped
2 tablespoons salsa
1 tablespoon low-fat sour cream

Top the tortilla with the beans and cheese. Microwave for about 90 seconds, or until the beans are warm and the cheese is melted. Top with the green pepper, tomato, salsa, and sour cream. Roll the tortilla and enjoy.

Per serving: 475 calories, 17 grams fat, 61 grams carbohydrate, 21 grams protein, 11 grams fiber

Ham Sandwich on Rye

SERVES 1

2 ounces lean ham
1 cup romaine lettuce leaves
2 slices rye bread*
1 tablespoon light mayonnaise*

Assemble the sandwich with the ingredients.

Per serving: 307 calories, 10 grams fat, 33 grams carbohydrate, 21 grams protein, 5 grams fiber

Watercress Black Bean Salad

SERVES 1

1 cup watercress
1 cup chopped fresh spinach
1 tomato, chopped
1/2 cup canned black beans, drained
1/2 cucumber, chopped
2 tablespoons regular Italian salad dressing*

Combine the watercress, spinach, tomato, black beans, and cucumber, and top with the dressing.

Per serving: 293 calories, 18 grams fat, 31 grams carbohydrate, 11 grams protein, 11 grams fiber

Spinach-Lentil Salad

SERVES 1

1 cup finely chopped red cabbage
1 cup chopped spinach
$1/2$ cup cooked lentils
$1/4$ cup chopped green onion
1 carrot, grated
2 tablespoons olive oil*
1 tablespoon balsamic vinegar

Toss the cabbage with the spinach, lentils, green onion, and carrot. Sprinkle on the oil and vinegar.

Per serving: 314 calories, 14 grams fat, 37 grams carbohydrate, 12 grams protein, 13 grams fiber

Cheesy Veggie Pile

SERVES 1

2 slices whole wheat bread
2 slices American cheese*
$1/2$ red pepper, cut in thin slices
1 cup watercress leaves, stems removed
2 tablespoons low-fat mayonnaise*

Assemble all the ingredients between 2 slices of bread.

Per serving: 319 calories, 14 grams fat, 39 grams carbohydrate, 12 grams protein, 14 grams fiber

Mandarin Orange Broil

SERVES 1

$1/2$ cup low-fat cottage cheese
$1/2$ English muffin*
$1/2$ cup canned mandarin oranges, drained
1 teaspoon sugar mixed with 1 teaspoon ground cinnamon

Place the cottage cheese on top of the English muffin half. Place the oranges on top of the cottage cheese and sprinkle with the sugar-cinnamon mixture. Place under a broiler until the top is bubbly and warm.

Per serving: 206 calories, 1.7 grams fat, 32 grams carbohydrate, 17 grams protein, 3 grams fiber

Carrot-Broccoli-Lemon Salad

SERVES 1

1 carrot, grated
$1/2$ cup frozen broccoli, thawed
1 tablespoon low-fat mayonnaise
1 tablespoon lemon juice

Combine the carrot and broccoli in a small bowl. In another small bowl, combine the mayonnaise and lemon juice. Pour over the vegetables and mix.

Per serving: 95 calories, 3 grams fat, 16 grams carbohydrate, 4 grams protein, 5 grams fiber

Tomato Turkey Stack

SERVES 1

2 slices whole wheat bread
2 ounces lean turkey breast*
2 large romaine lettuce leaves
2 thick slices tomato
1 tablespoon light mayonnaise

Assemble the sandwich with the ingredients.

Per serving: 353 calories, 12 grams fat, 31 grams carbohydrate, 32 grams protein, 5 grams fiber

Sweet Pepper Medley

SERVES 1

$1/2$ each: sweet green pepper, sweet red pepper, sweet yellow pepper, chopped
1 tablespoon Italian dressing
$1/4$ cup finely chopped fresh cilantro
2 cups baby spinach leaves

Combine the chopped peppers in a bowl with the Italian dressing and mix well. Add the cilantro and serve over the bed of spinach leaves.

Per serving: 111 calories, 8 grams fat, 11 grams carbohydrate, 3 grams protein, 4 grams fiber

Tuna Tomato Stack

SERVES I

3 ounces tuna fish packed in water, drained
2 tablespoons light mayonnaise
2 slices whole wheat bread*
2 romaine lettuce leaves
2 thick slices tomato

Combine the tuna fish and mayonnaise. Spread the mixture on 1 slice of bread and top with the tomatoes, lettuce, and the other slice of bread.

Per sandwich: 331 calories, 9 grams fat, 36 grams carbohydrate, 29 grams protein, 6 grams fiber

Confetti Rice Salad

SERVES 3 (ABOUT 2⅔ CUPS PER SERVING)

Salad:
I large carrot, grated (about I cup)
I green bell pepper, finely chopped
I yellow bell pepper, finely chopped
I red bell pepper, finely chopped
4 green onions, finely chopped (about I cup)
I ½ cups cooked brown rice
I cup cooked black beans (use canned, but rinse and drain well)
I cup dark red kidney beans (use canned, but rinse and drain well)

Sauce:
2 tablespoons extra-virgin olive oil
¼ cup plus 2 tablespoons balsamic vinegar
2 tablespoons sugar
about ¾ teaspoon coarsely ground black pepper, or to taste

Place all the salad ingredients in a large serving bowl. Mix the sauce ingredients in a small cup, pour over the salad ingredients, and toss to mix. Chill at least 1 hour.

Per serving: 456 calories, 11 grams fat, 76 grams carbohydrate, 14 grams protein, 14 grams fiber

Black Bean Salad

SERVES 1

1/4 cup chopped green onions
6 cherry tomatoes, halved
1/2 cup cooked black beans
1/2 cup cooked lentils
2 tablespoons Italian salad dressing
1 cup chopped romaine lettuce
1 cup chopped radicchio

In a small bowl, combine the onions, tomatoes, black beans, lentils, and dressing. Toss to combine. Mix the radicchio and romaine lettuce on a plate and top with the black bean mixture.

Per serving: 413 calories, 18 grams fat, 52 grams carbohydrate, 20 grams protein, 18 grams fiber

Pita Stuffed with Peanut Butter and Banana

SERVES 1

1 banana, thinly sliced
2 tablespoons chunky peanut butter
1/2 whole wheat pita*

In a small bowl, mix the banana slices and peanut butter. Stuff into the pita.

Per serving: 382 calories, 17 grams fat, 53 grams carbohydrate, 12 grams protein, 7 grams fiber

Kris's Split Pea Soup

SERVES 8

1 small ham bone
4 medium onions, coarsely chopped
4 beef bouillon cubes
3 tablespoons reduced-sodium beef bouillon granules
4 bay leaves
4½ cups raw split peas (2 one-pound bags)
11 cups water
½ teaspoon black pepper
2–3 cloves garlic, minced

Remove the fat from the ham bone. Combine all the ingredients in a large stock pot, bring to a boil, lower the heat, and simmer for 2 hours. Remove bay leaves before serving.

Per serving (⅛ of recipe): 471 calories, 2 grams fat, 79 grams carbohydrate, 37 grams protein, 11 grams fiber

FOR DINNER

Grilled Vegetable Medley

SERVES 1

½ green pepper, cut in strips
½ sweet red pepper, cut in strips
½ yellow pepper, cut in strips
¼ eggplant, thinly sliced and each slice quartered
1 tablespoon olive oil
2 tablespoons balsamic vinegar
½ cup fresh rosemary leaves
garlic powder and freshly ground pepper to taste

Combine the peppers and eggplant. Toss with the oil, vinegar, rosemary, garlic powder, and pepper. Place in a grill basket and grill until the eggplant is tender.

Per serving: 289 calories, 16 grams fat, 34 grams carbohydrate, 4 grams protein, 7 grams fiber

Sour Cream and Chives Baked Potato

SERVES 1

1 tablespoon low-fat sour cream*
2 tablespoons chopped chives
1 medium-sized baked potato

Mix the sour cream and chives. Top the potato with the mixture.

Per serving: 174 calories, 3 grams fat, 33 grams carbohydrate, 5 grams protein, 3 grams fiber

Lemon, Basil, and Ginger Tofu Stir-Fry with Spinach Rotini

SERVES 4

Stir-Fry:
2 tablespoons canola oil
4 cloves garlic, chopped
1-inch piece of fresh ginger, peeled and diced
2 cups chopped red onions
3 cups bite-sized broccoli pieces
1 red bell pepper, cut in strips
1 yellow bell pepper, cut in strips
1 green bell pepper, cut in strips
freshly ground black pepper to taste
3/4 teaspoon salt
1 cup chopped fresh basil leaves
2 tablespoons freshly squeezed lemon juice
2 teaspoons sugar
2 teaspoons cornstarch mixed in 2 tablespoons water until smooth
1 package (12.3 ounces) extra-firm lite tofu, cut into bite-sized squares.

Pasta:
4 cups cooked rotini*
1 tablespoon canola oil
1 clove garlic, chopped
1 pound fresh spinach leaves, chopped
2 tablespoons freshly squeezed lemon juice

To prepare the stir-fry: heat the oil, garlic, and ginger over low heat and sauté for 3 to 5 minutes. Turn the heat to high. Add the onions and broccoli. Stir-fry for 3 minutes, adding water by the tablespoonful as needed for enough moisture for cooking (this is called stir-sizzling).

Add the bell pepper strips and lower the heat to medium. Stir in the black pepper, salt, basil, lemon juice, and sugar. Gently stir in the cornstarch paste until the liquid thickens.

Reduce the heat to low and fold in the tofu. Cover and let the tofu heat through for 3 or 4 minutes.

To prepare the pasta: in the same pot in which you cooked the rotini, heat the oil over low heat. Sauté the garlic for 3 to 5 minutes. Turn the heat to medium high. Add the spinach and lemon juice, and mix thoroughly. Cover and let the spinach wilt for 2 or 3 minutes. Remove from the heat, stir in the cooked rotini, and toss to mix. Serve the tofu vegetable mixture over the pasta.

Per serving ($^1/_4$ of recipe): 443 calories, 13 grams fat, 66 grams carbohydrate, 20 grams protein, 10 grams fiber

Juicy Grilled Hamburger with Vidalia Onion on Whole Wheat Bun

SERVES 1

3 ounces very lean ground beef, formed into a patty
1 whole-grain bun
1 thick slice Vidalia onion
1 thick slice tomato
1 tablespoon ketchup

Grill or broil the patty. Place on the bun and top with the onion, tomato, and ketchup.

Per serving: 300 calories, 9 grams fat, 24 grams carbohydrate, 30 grams protein, 2 grams fiber

Chicken Stir-Fry

SERVES 1

2 ounces chicken breast, cut in strips
2 cups sliced raw red cabbage
1 cup asparagus pieces
$^1/_4$ cup chopped Vidalia onion
1 tablespoon olive oil

Stir-fry the chicken, cabbage, asparagus, and onion in the oil for 8 to 10 minutes or until chicken is thoroughly cooked.

Per serving: 312 calories, 18 grams fat, 17 grams carbohydrate, 22 grams protein, 7 grams fiber

Roasted Red Pepper, Salmon, and Quinoa Salad

SERVES 5

Marinade:
$\frac{1}{2}$ cup cilantro leaves
2 tablespoons balsamic vinegar
$\frac{1}{2}$ teaspoon sugar

4 ounces salmon fillet

Salad:
$\frac{1}{2}$ cup raw quinoa
1 teaspoon olive oil
$\frac{1}{4}$ teaspoon salt
freshly ground black pepper to taste
1 tablespoon balsamic vinegar
$\frac{1}{2}$ teaspoon sugar
$\frac{1}{2}$ cup chopped cilantro leaves
4 ounces asparagus, cut on the diagonal into 1 inch pieces
$\frac{1}{2}$ small jar (7.25 ounces) roasted red peppers (water packed) or 1 roasted red pepper, cut into strips
$\frac{1}{2}$ cup chopped red onion
1 generous cup chopped romaine lettuce

To make the marinade: place the cilantro leaves, vinegar, and sugar in a mini food processor and process until the leaves are finely minced. Alternatively, mince the cilantro leaves by hand and blend with the vinegar and sugar. Place the marinade in a shallow glass dish. Place the salmon fillet on top of the marinade, skin side up. Marinate for at least 4 hours or overnight in the refrigerator.

To prepare the salad: boil 1 cup of water in a small saucepan. Add the quinoa, oil, and salt. Lower the heat and simmer for 15 to 20 minutes. Remove from the heat and stir in the pepper, vinegar, sugar, cilantro leaves, asparagus, and red onion. Chill for at least 2 hours, but overnight is fine.

Just before dinner, grill the marinated salmon, skin side down, for 4 to 8 minutes, depending on grill temperature; alternatively, broil until done. Remove the skin and slice into strips.

Build the salad: place the lettuce on a plate. Top with the quinoa-vegetable mixture, the salmon strips, and finally the red pepper strips.

Per serving ($\frac{1}{5}$ of recipe): 576 calories, 9 grams fat, 85 grams carbohydrate, 39 grams protein, 15 grams fiber

Black Bean, Barley, and Leek Soup

SERVES 5

1 tablespoon extra-virgin olive oil
4 cloves garlic, minced
3 leeks, cleaned and chopped
1 cup dry black beans
1 cup dry medium barley
8 cups water
1 teaspoon freshly ground black pepper
1 tablespoon plus 1 teaspoon beef bouillon granules
2 tablespoons very low sodium beef bouillon granules
8 ounces kale, stems removed and chopped
6 ounces portobello mushrooms, sliced and quartered

Heat the oil with the garlic over low heat. Add the leeks and sauté for 5 to 7 minutes, or until the leeks are wilted.

Add the beans, barley, water, pepper, and bouillon. Simmer for 1 hour; the mixture should have a slight bubble.

Add the kale and mushrooms, and simmer 15 minutes more.

Per serving ($\frac{1}{5}$ of recipe): 362 calories, 5 grams fat, 67 grams carbohydrate, 16 grams protein, 14 grams fiber

Hearty Chicken Tabbouleh Salad

SERVES 1

Sauce:
2 teaspoons extra-virgin olive oil
2 tablespoons fresh lemon juice
1 clove garlic, minced
$\frac{1}{4}$ teaspoon salt
1 teaspoon sugar
$\frac{1}{4}$ teaspoon coarsely ground pepper

Salad:
1 cup cooked bulgur wheat, cooled
1 ripe medium tomato, chopped
2 green onions, chopped ($\frac{1}{2}$ cup)
3 ounces cooked chicken breast, cooled and chopped
1 cup chopped romaine lettuce

In a small mixing bowl, blend the sauce ingredients. Add the bulgur and toss with a fork. Add the tomato, onions, and chicken, and toss gently to combine. Place the lettuce on a dinner plate; and top with the salad.

Per serving: 449 calories, 13 grams fat, 51 grams carbohydrate, 33 grams protein, 11 grams fiber

Rosemary-Roasted Winter Veggies and Chicken

SERVES 4

1 pound acorn squash, cut in half and seeds removed
1 large sweet potato, peeled and sliced into 4 pieces
4 parsnips, peeled and quartered
1 red onion, peeled and quartered
12 ounces skinless, boneless chicken breast
2 tablespoons olive oil
2 tablespoons balsamic vinegar
1 teaspoon freshly ground black pepper
1 teaspoon garlic powder
1/3 cup coarsely chopped fresh rosemary

Combine all the ingredients in a clay roaster and toss to mix. Cover tightly and bake at 350 degrees for 1 to 1½ hours, or until all the vegetables are fork-tender.

Per serving (1/4 of recipe): 469 calories, 11 grams fat, 63 grams carbohydrate, 31 grams protein, 11 grams fiber

Turkey Burger on Bun with Sliced Vidalia Onion

SERVES 1

4 ounces lean raw ground turkey
garlic powder to taste
Black pepper to taste
2 thick slices Vidalia onion
2 teaspoons fat-free mayonnaise
1 whole wheat bun

Form the turkey into a patty and season with garlic and pepper. Grill or broil until well done. Place on the bun and add the onion slices and mayonnaise.

Per burger on bun: 256 calories, 4 grams fat, 24 grams carbohydrate, 32 grams protein, 3 grams fiber

Steamed Veggies with Basil and Olive Oil

SERVES 1

1/2 cup cauliflower florets
1/2 cup broccoli florets
2 teaspoons extra-virgin olive oil
1/4 cup chopped fresh basil

Toss the vegetables with the oil and basil. Place in a microwave-safe container and cook on high for approximately 5 minutes, or until the vegetables are crisp-tender.

Per serving: 104 calories, 9 grams fat, 5 grams carbohydrate, 2.3 grams protein, 3 grams fiber

Soy-Orange-Marinated Red Snapper

SERVES 1

1/4 cup orange juice
1 teaspoon extra-virgin olive oil
1 tablespoon soy sauce
4 ounces red snapper fillet

Combine the orange juice, oil, and soy sauce in a shallow container. Place the fish in the marinade for at least 2 hours; overnight is best. Remove the fish from the marinade. Broil on each side for 3 to 4 minutes.

Per serving: 212 calories, 10 grams fat, 5 grams carbohydrate, 23 grams protein, 0 fiber

Creamed Chicken on Toast

SERVES 4

1 pound skinless, boneless chicken breast, cut into 1-inch pieces
10 pearl onions
3 tablespoons reduced-sodium chicken bouillon granules
2 cups chopped green bell peppers
1 cup skim milk
1 can condensed cream of chicken soup
1/2 cup low-fat sour cream
4 slices whole wheat bread or toast

Coat a nonstick pan with vegetable oil spray and heat over medium-high heat. Add the chicken pieces, onions, and bouillon granules, and stir-fry until the chicken is cooked, about 10 to 12 minutes. Add the green peppers, milk, soup, and sour cream. Mix well with a whisk and heat through. Serve 1/4 of the mixture over 1 slice of bread or toast for each serving.

Per serving (1/4 of recipe): 440 calories; 10 grams fat, 40 grams carbohydrate, 46 grams protein, 4 grams fiber

Chicken-Veggie Stir-Fry over Linguine

SERVES 2

1 tablespoon dark sesame oil
2 cloves garlic, minced
¼ cup chopped Vidalia onion
8 ounces boneless, skinless chicken breast, cut for stir-fry
2 cups broccoli florets
1 sweet red bell pepper, thinly sliced
freshly ground black pepper to taste
1 cup cooked linguine

Heat the oil over low heat. Add the garlic and onion, and sauté for 5 minutes.

Raise the heat and add the chicken. Stir-fry for 5 minutes, adding water by the tablespoon as necessary.

Add the broccoli and red pepper, and stir-fry briefly until the chicken is thoroughly cooked and the vegetables are crisp-tender.

Season with the pepper and serve over the linguine, ½ cup per person.

Per serving (½ of recipe): 341 calories, 11 grams fat, 28 grams carbohydrate, 33 grams protein, 5 grams fiber

Parsnip Whipped Potatoes

SERVES 8

1½ pounds Yukon Gold potatoes (about 3), peeled and cut into
   1-inch cubes
1 pound parsnips (about 3), peeled and cut into 1-inch pieces
kosher salt
2 tablespoons unsalted butter, softened
2 tablespoons heavy cream
¼ cup 2% milk
¼ teaspoon freshly grated nutmeg
a few grinds black pepper

Place the potatoes and parsnips in a 4-quart pot and cover with water seasoned with a pinch of salt. Bring to a boil, reduce the heat, cover, and simmer for 20 to 30 minutes, or until very tender. Drain and return the parsnips and potatoes to the pot.

Mash the hot parsnips and potatoes with a potato masher or a handheld mixer. Beat in the butter.

In a small saucepan, heat the cream and milk until hot but not boiling. Add to the mashed parsnips and potatoes, and beat until fluffy. Season with the nutmeg, salt, and pepper.

Per serving ($^1/_8$ of recipe): 163 calories, 4 grams fat, 29 grams carbohydrate, 3 grams protein, 4 grams fiber

(Recipe courtesy of Larry P. Forgione, chef and proprietor of An American Place, Rose Hill, and The Coach House in New York City, and The Beekman 1766 Tavern at the Beekman Arms in Rhinebeck, New York.)

Grilled Asparagus and Leeks

SERVES 6

1 pound fresh leeks
1 pound fresh asparagus
1 tablespoon olive oil
kosher salt and freshly ground pepper

Cut off the roots of the leeks, leaving as much of the white part as possible. Cut off the green tops just at the point where the stem branches into leaves. Wash thoroughly under cold running water. Be careful to remove all traces of grit.

Bring about 2 inches of salted water to a boil in a large skillet. Lay the leeks in the pan and cook for 6 to 7 minutes. The point of a sharp knife should easily pass through the leeks. Remove from the water and shock in iced water to stop further cooking. Set aside.

Wash, snap off coarse lower stems, and peel the asparagus. Blanch in salted boiling water and shock to stop cooking. Set aside.

Prepare a charcoal, wood, or gas grill, or preheat the broiler. Brush the leeks and asparagus with the olive oil and season with salt and pepper. Place on the grill (or under the broiler) and cook until tender, taking care not to burn. Serve immediately.

Per serving ($^1/_6$ of recipe): 83 calories, 3 grams fat, 14 grams carbohydrate, 3 grams protein, 3 grams fiber

(Recipe courtesy of Larry P. Forgione, chef and proprietor of An American Place, Rose Hill, and The Coach House in New York City, and The Beekman 1766 Tavern at the Beekman Arms in Rhinebeck, New York.)

Shrimp Slaw with Jicama, Pineapple and Watercress

SERVES 6

3 cups watercress
8 ounces fresh pineapple, about a quarter of a pineapple
24 poached shrimp, cooked, peeled, and deveined
2 cups peeled and thinly sliced jicama
I cup thinly sliced red bell pepper, cut into strips
juice of 2 limes
2 tablespoons chopped fresh cilantro
I ½ teaspoons chili oil
kosher salt and freshly ground pepper to taste

Wash the watercress and pick the tender branches from the main stems. Arrange these branches in the center of the plate to make a nest. Discard the stems.

Using a sharp knife, peel the pineapple and slice it thinly, saving any juices. Cut the slices into strips.

Cut the shrimp into thin strips and place in a bowl with the pineapple, jicama slices, red pepper slices, pineapple juice, lime juice, cilantro, and chili oil. Toss and season to taste with salt and pepper. Let stand for 10 minutes.

Using a slotted spoon, place the shrimp salad over the watercress and drizzle with the remaining dressing.

Per serving (⅙ of recipe): 97 calories, 4 grams fat, 11 grams carbohydrate, 6 grams protein, 3 grams fiber

(Recipe courtesy of Larry P. Forgione, chef and proprietor of An American Place, Rose Hill, and The Coach House in New York City, and The Beekman 1766 Tavern at the Beekman Arms in Rhinebeck, New York.)

Herb-Seared Day Boat Cod with Fresh Stewed Tomatoes

SERVES 6

Fresh stewed tomatoes:
2 teaspoons extra virgin olive oil
2 teaspoons minced garlic
2 teaspoons chopped shallots
2 pints small ripe cherry tomatoes, red plums, or golden plums
I tablespoon red wine vinegar
freshly ground black pepper, to taste

Cod:
6 cod fillets (5 ounces each), skinned and boned
salt and freshly ground black pepper to taste
4 tablespoons chopped fresh herbs such as chervil, tarragon, basil, and oregano
½ tablespoon olive oil
2 tablespoons fresh lemon juice

Cut each tomato in half.

Heat 1 teaspoon of oil in a nonstick pan. Add the garlic and shallots, and slowly cook for 1–2 minutes.

Add the halved tomatoes and season generously with pepper. Stir and cook for just a minute.

Deglaze the pan with the vinegar and bring to a simmer. Remove from the heat and stir in the other teaspoon of oil.

Season the cod fillets with salt and pepper. Sprinkle each fillet evenly with lemon juice and herbs, pressing them into the flesh with your fingers.

Heat the olive oil in a nonstick skillet over high heat. Lay the fillets in the skillet, herb side down, and cook for 2 or 3 minutes. Lower the heat to medium-high and carefully turn the fillets over. Cook 2 or 3 minutes longer, until the fish is cooked through. Place the fillets on plates and spoon the stewed tomatoes over the cod.

Per serving (¹⁄₆ of recipe): 161 calories, 4 grams fat, 3 grams carbohydrate, 28 grams protein, 1 gram fiber

(Recipe courtesy of Larry P. Forgione, chef and proprietor of An American Place, Rose Hill, and The Coach House in New York City, and The Beekman 1766 Tavern at the Beekman Arms in Rhinebeck, New York.)

Breast of Chicken with Braised White Beans and Arugula

SERVES 4

1 tablespoon extra-virgin olive oil
4 (6-ounce) skinless, boneless chicken breasts
kosher salt and freshly ground pepper to taste
1 cup sliced onion
2 teaspoons minced garlic
2 cups cooked or canned and drained white beans, such as cannellini or Great Northern
1 tablespoon fresh thyme
2 cups arugula
1 cup homemade chicken broth or low-sodium canned broth (skimmed of all fat)

In a large nonstick skillet, heat the olive oil. Season the chicken breasts with salt and pepper and sear them over high heat for 2 or 3 minutes on each side. Remove the chicken from the pan and set aside to keep warm.

Add the onion, garlic, white beans, and fresh thyme, and sauté the pan ingredients for 2 to 3 minutes. Return the chicken to the pan and add the chicken broth. Continue to cook until the liquid is reduced by half, turning the chicken one time. Stir in the arugula.

Place the chicken breasts in the center of your plates and spoon the bean and arugula mixture over the chicken. Serve immediately.

Per serving: 379 calories, 10 grams fat, 19 grams carbohydrate, 50 grams protein, 5 grams fiber

(Recipe courtesy of Larry P. Forgione, chef and proprietor of An American Place, Rose Hill, and The Coach House in New York City, and The Beekman 1766 Tavern at the Beekman Arms in Rhinebeck, New York.)

Penne with Grilled Chicken and Forest Mushrooms

SERVES 6

12 ounces dried penne
2 (8-ounce) boned and skinned chicken breast halves
12 shiitake or other wild mushrooms
1 red onion, peeled and cut into ½-inch slices
1 tablespoon extra-virgin olive oil
kosher salt and freshly ground pepper to taste
2 teaspoons minced garlic
1 large ripe tomato, peeled, seeded, and chopped
16 snow peas, cut at an angle into lengthwise strips
1½ teaspoons chopped fresh marjoram
1 tablespoon chopped parsley
1 cup homemade chicken broth or low-sodium canned broth (skimmed of all fat)

Prepare a charcoal, wood, or gas grill, or preheat the broiler.

Bring a large saucepan of water to a boil and cook the penne for 10 to 12 minutes. Drain and set aside.

Brush the chicken breasts, mushrooms, and onion slices with some of the oil and sprinkle with salt and freshly ground pepper to taste.

Grill the chicken over medium-hot coals on each side for about 3 minutes on each side for medium rare to medium meat. Grill the mushrooms for 1 minute to a side and the onion slices for 3 minutes to a side. Set all the vegetables aside to cool to room temperature.

Using a sharp knife, cut the chicken breasts and mushrooms into thin strips. Cut each onion ring in half. Briefly sauté the garlic, chopped tomato, snow peas, and herbs in a large skillet. Add the chicken, mushrooms, and onions and cook over medium-high heat for about 1 minute. Add the pasta and chicken broth, and bring to a boil. Ladle into shallow soup bowls.

Per serving (⅙ of recipe): 374 calories, 6 grams fat, 54 grams carbohydrate, 30 grams protein, 8 grams fiber

(Recipe courtesy of Larry P. Forgione, chef and proprietor of An American Place, Rose Hill, and The Coach House in New York City, and The Beekman 1766 Tavern at the Beekman Arms in Rhinebeck, New York.)

FOR DESSERT

Raspberry Cheesecake

SERVES 8

Cheesecake:

1 (8-ounce) package low-fat cream cheese at room temperature
1 (8-ounce) package nonfat cream cheese at room temperature
1 (32-ounce) carton plain nonfat yogurt, strained into yogurt cheese
2 eggs
3/4 cup granulated sugar
1 tablespoon vanilla extract
3 tablespoons cornstarch

Sauce:

2 cups fresh raspberries, divided
1 tablespoon granulated sugar

To make the cheesecake: Preheat the oven to 325 degrees. Beat together both packages of cream cheese until completely smooth. Add the yogurt cheese and beat until smooth. Add the eggs, sugar, vanilla, and cornstarch. Beat for 3 minutes on high, until smooth.

Coat a 9-inch deep dish pie plate with vegetable oil spray. Transfer the cheesecake mixture to the pie plate. Bake for 50 to 60 minutes, or until a knife inserted in the middle comes out clean. Chill.

To make the sauce: Set aside 1 cup of berries. Place the remaining cup of berries in a mini food processor with the sugar. Process until smooth.

To serve, place 1/8 of the sauce over each slice of cheesecake and top with the whole berries.

Per serving (1/8 of cheesecake and 1/8 of sauce): 269 calories, 6 grams fat, 40 grams carbohydrate, 14 grams protein, 2 grams fiber

Peach Creamsicle Sundae with Marion Blackberry Fruit Perfect

SERVES 4

¹/₂ pint fresh peach sorbet (Ciao Bella)
¹/₂ pint low-fat vanilla frozen yogurt (Ciao Bella)
¹/₂ cup Marion Blackberry Fruit Perfect (American Spoon Foods)

Scoop both the peach sorbet and the vanilla yogurt into 4 sundae bowls. Top each with 2 tablespoons of the Marion Blackberry Fruit Perfect.

Per serving (¹/₄ of recipe): 105 calories, 1 gram fat, 22 grams carbohydrate, 3 grams protein, 0 fiber

(Recipe courtesy of Larry P. Forgione, chef and proprietor of An American Place, Rose Hill, and The Coach House in New York City, and The Beekman 1766 Tavern at the Beekman Arms in Rhinebeck, New York.)

Warm Pear and Blueberry Granola Crisp with Maple Yogurt

SERVES 6

3 ripe pears
1 pint fresh blueberries
¹/₂ tablespoon unsalted butter
2 tablespoons brown sugar
pinch of ground cinnamon
pinch of nutmeg
1¹/₃ cups low-fat granola
¹/₂ cup low-fat yogurt with 2 tablespoons pure maple syrup

Preheat the oven to 425 degrees. Peel and core the pears and cut into eighths.

Rinse the blueberries, discarding any that are bad and pulling off and discarding the stems.

In a large nonstick skillet, melt the butter over medium heat. Add the pears and cook for 3 or 4 minutes, stirring occasionally. Add the brown sugar, cinnamon, and nutmeg, and cook another minute. Add the blueberries and stir. Continue to cook, stirring occasionally, for 2 or 3 minutes.

Spoon the fruit mixture into a casserole dish and top with the granola.

Bake for 10 minutes. Spoon into 6 serving bowls and top with the maple yogurt.

Per serving (¹/₆ of recipe): 197 calories, 6 grams fat, 36 grams carbohydrate, 4 grams protein, 5 grams fiber

(Recipe courtesy of Larry P. Forgione, chef and proprietor of An American Place, Rose Hill, and The Coach House in New York City, and The Beekman 1766 Tavern at the Beekman Arms in Rhinebeck, New York.)

Old-Fashioned Apple and Fresh Raspberry Cobbler

SERVES 8

Fruit:

3/4 cup granulated sugar

2 tablespoons quick-cooking tapioca

1 cup apple cider

1 cup fresh raspberries

2 tablespoons applejack (apple brandy)

1 tablespoon grated fresh ginger

zest of 1 lemon, grated

6 tart apples, such as Macoun or Northern Spy, peeled, cored, and sliced

Topping:

2 large egg yolks

1/3 cup granulated sugar

1 teaspoon pure vanilla extract

2 large egg whites

1/4 cup all-purpose flour

confectioners' sugar, for dusting

Preheat the oven to 350 degrees and butter a 2½ quart baking dish.

To prepare the fruit: combine the sugar and tapioca in a large saucepan and stir in the apple cider. Cook over medium heat, stirring until the sugar dissolves. Stir in the applejack, ginger, lemon zest, and apples. Raise the heat to high and bring to a boil. Lower the heat to a simmer, cover, and cook for about 4 minutes, until the apples are slightly softened. Fold in the raspberries and spoon the fruit into the baking dish.

To prepare the topping: beat the egg yolks and sugar with an electric mixer for about 3 or 4 minutes, until thick and lemon-colored. Stir in the vanilla.

In another bowl, using clean beaters, beat the egg whites with an electric mixer until soft peaks form. Fold the flour into the whites. Fold the whites into the egg yolk mixture.

Pour the topping over the fruit, spreading it gently with a rubber spatula, cover the surface. Bake, uncovered, for 20 to 25 minutes, until the topping is golden brown and begins to pull away from the sides of the pan.

Let the cobbler cool slightly. Dust with the confectioners' sugar and serve warm.

Per serving (⅛ of recipe): 237 calories, 2 grams fat, 53 grams carbohydrate, 3 grams protein, 4 grams fiber

(Recipe courtesy of Larry P. Forgione, chef and proprietor of An American Place, Rose Hill, and The Coach House in New York City, and The Beekman 1766 Tavern at the Beekman Arms in Rhinebeck, New York.)

c h a p t e r

5

On Your Own: Creating Your Own Menus and Eating Out

Use our menus as often as you want—or create your own. Another possibility is to use a mix of our menus and your own; this gives you the most variety and flexibility. Using the same format of our menus in chapter 4, we've provided the guidelines for you to create your own. Use the chart below the same way that you do the prepared menus. Find the calorie level you want to follow and then read down the column to find the number of servings required for each food. The following pages have information on what portion sizes these servings represent.

A Generic Prototype for Creating Your Own Menus

Food	1,300 calories	1,400 calories	1,500 calories	1,600 calories	1,700 calories
BREAKFAST (NUMBER OF SERVINGS)					
Protein food	1	1	1	1	1
Grain food	1	2	2	2	2
Fruit	1	1	1	1	1
Dairy food	1	1	1	1	1
Added fat	1	1	1	1	1

Food	1,300 calories	1,400 calories	1,500 calories	1,600 calories	1,700 calories
LUNCH (NUMBER OF SERVINGS)					
Protein food	2	2	2	2	3
Grain food	1	1	2	2	2
Vegetable	2	2	2	2	2
Fruit	1	1	1	1	1
Dairy food	1	1	1	1	1
Added fat	2	2	2	2	2
DINNER (NUMBER OF SERVINGS)					
Protein food	3	3	3	3	4
Grain food	1	1	1	2	2
Vegetable	3	3	3	3	3
Fruit	1	1	1	1	1
Added fat	2	2	2	2	2
SNACKS (NUMBER OF SERVINGS)					
Grain food	0	0	1	1	1
Vegetable	2	2	2	2	2
Fruit	1	2	2	3	3
Dairy food	1	1	1	1	1

What Is in a Serving?

Fruit Portion Sizes. In general, one piece of fruit counts as one serving. Alternatively, ½ cup of berries and 1 cup of cut-up melon constitute a serving. Calories vary by fruit, but these guidelines work well enough without your having to look up actual calories.

Grain Food Portion Sizes. In general, the following sizes constitute one serving of a grain: ½ cup of cooked grain, rice or pasta; 1 slice of bread; ½ of most bagels (although bagels from bagel stores are so large that ⅓ of such bagels is one serving).

Vegetable Portion Sizes. In general, ½ cup of a cooked vegetable and 1 cup of a raw vegetable constitute a serving. Starchy vegetables, including peas, corn, potatoes, and sweet potatoes, should be counted under grain foods.

Dairy Food Portion Sizes. Choose nonfat dairy foods when possible. One serving is equivalent to: 8 ounces nonfat milk or yogurt or low-fat yogurt. Note that other dairy foods are listed under *Protein* and *Added Fat.*

Protein Portion Sizes. As you create your own menus, you'll need some guidelines about protein foods. Under protein foods we've listed a certain number of servings, but serving size varies by the type of protein food chosen. One serving is equivalent to:

- ½ cup cooked beans, 4 ounces light tofu or 3 ounces tempeh
- 1 ounce of skinless chicken or turkey breast; also extra-lean ground turkey breast (the package must be marked extra-lean)
- 1 ounce of fatty fish, such as salmon, mackerel, or tuna
- 2 ounces of lean fish such as cod, shrimp, lobster, crab, or canned tuna (in water or brine)
- 1 ounce of very lean beef or pork
- 1 whole egg
- 1 ounce low-fat cheese (5 grams or less per serving) or 2 ounces nonfat cheese

Added Fat Portion Sizes. You'll also need guidance for using added fats. Remember that you can use added fats; they make your diet palatable, enjoyable, and satisfying. Just account for them. You can either use Table 4, page 146, which gives specific fat grams, or you can use the following general guidelines for serving sizes. Use added fats in food preparation, as a condiment, or, in the case of nuts, as a food. Each of the following food amounts counts as one added fat serving:

- 1 teaspoon margarine, butter, or cooking oil
- 2 teaspoons reduced-fat margarine
- 1 tablespoon reduced-fat mayonnaise or reduced-fat Miracle Whip
- 1 teaspoon regular mayonnaise or Miracle Whip
- 1 tablespoon regular or 2 tablespoons low-fat cream cheese
- 2 tablespoons regular or 3 tablespoons low-fat sour cream
- 1 tablespoon nuts or peanut butter
- 4 chocolate kisses

Keeping Records: Your Personal Food Diary

As you create your own menus, and even as you use ours, it is important to keep careful track of what you actually eat. Use this food diary to record what you eat, to calculate total calories, and to track fat grams for each meal so that you don't exceed the 20-gram maximum. Our chart, which can be photocopied, is also a useful tool for planning your daily menus.

My Food Diary

Meal	Food Eaten	Serving Size	Number of Calories	Number of Fat Grams	Total Number of Fat Grams for the Meal (Not to Exceed 20 Grams)
Breakfast					
Lunch					
Dinner					
Snacks					
Total Daily Fat and Calories					

Monitoring Fat: Guidelines and Tables

Because Xenical works best when you limit fat to about 30 percent of your daily calories—and when you eat no more than about 20 grams of fat at any one time—it is extremely important to understand where you pick up fat grams. If you are using our menus, you know they fall within this range. If you are creating your own menus, simply tally up all the fat grams you eat (including those used in preparing food) and stop at 20 grams per meal. Remember, snacks have to be very low in fat while you are taking Xenical because the drug has a limited time of action and does not continue to work long after a meal is eaten.

To help you keep a watchful eye on your intake, here are the main sources of fat in the diet. Following this information you will find some useful fat-counter tables for the different food groups.

Added Fats. There are two types of added fats: those you add in cooking such as oils and creams, and those you add as a garnish or condiment, which include sour cream, cream cheese, butter, and margarine. Refer to Table 4 for the number of fat grams in common foods in these categories. You'll have to limit the amount of fat you use in cooking, which is why we've provided many fabulous low-fat cooking ideas later in this chapter.

Dairy Foods. From yogurt to milk to cheese, dairy foods are often a significant source of fat. In many cases you can find a low-fat or a non-fat substitute to dramatically cut the fat grams. Refer to Table 5 for comparisons.

Protein Foods (see Tables 6 and 7). Choosing protein foods carefully is one of the most powerful ways to cut fat grams. Overall, vegetable sources of protein, such as black beans and lentils, are the lowest fat source of protein; fish is generally the next lowest; after that, poultry, beef, and pork have more fat grams for the amount of protein they provide. Sausages, regular luncheon meats, and bacon generally contain prohibitive amounts of fat.

Nuts and Seeds. Peanuts, soy nuts, and sunflower seeds are among the nuts and seeds that fit into a healthy diet—as long as you account for their fat grams. Refer to Table 8 for fat grams per serving. Because these foods are relatively high in fat, you'll have to include them in meals and not snacks (remember, snacks should be low-fat while using Xenical).

Convenience Packaged Foods. Boxed macaroni and cheese, prepared pasta mixes, and boxed main courses often contain too many fat grams to make them suitable for dieters (or for anyone who is health conscious). If you want to use these foods, read the labels carefully and take note of the portion sizes. You'll have to tally the fat grams in these individual foods rather than rely on generic guidelines.

Frozen Dinners and Entrees. There is a huge variation here in fat grams and suitability for lower fat eating. Again, the best advice is to read the labels carefully and tally the fat grams.

Grain-Based Foods (see Table 9). Since they come from nature, grain foods are naturally low in fat and suitable for lower fat eating. Brown rice, quinoa, and barley are great foods that supply lots of complex carbohydrates, nutrients, fiber, and energy—and for only a few fat grams. But you have to start paying attention to fat grams when these foods are processed. Most crackers, for example, are notoriously high in fat grams, as are cookies and croissants. On the other hand, some processed grain foods such as bread and pasta are very low in fat so long as you don't top the bread with fat, such as margarine, or cover the pasta with a high-fat sauce. Try to choose whole-grain bread, rice, breakfast cereal, and pasta whenever possible to get the maximum nutrition for your money. Be aware, though, that granola cereals can be quite high in fat, so always read labels and count fat grams accordingly.

TABLE 4
Fat Grams in Added Fats

Food	Calories	Protein (g)	Total Fat (g)	Saturated Fat (g)	Cholesterol (mg)
Olive oil, 1 tsp.	40	0	4	1	0
Sour cream, regular, 1 tsp.	11	0	1	1	2
Sour cream, low-fat, 1 tsp.	7	0	0	0	2
Sour cream, fat-free, 1 tsp.	5	0	0	0	0
Cream cheese, regular, 1 tsp.	17	0	2	1	5
Cream cheese, low-fat, 1 tsp.	12	1	1	1	3
Cream cheese, fat-free, 1 tsp.	5	1	0	0	0
Butter, 1 tsp.	34	0	4	2	10
Stick margarine, 1 tsp.	34	0	4	1	0
Tub margarine, 1 tsp.	34	0	4	1	0
Light margarine, 1 tsp.	17	0	2	0	0
Mayonnaise, 1 tsp.	19	0	2	0	1
Mayonnaise, light, 1 tsp.	12	0	1	0	1
Mayonnaise, fat-free, 1 tsp.	3	0	0	0	0
Salad dressing, regular, 1 tsp.	23	0	3	0	0
Salad dressing, light, 1 tsp.	5	0	0	0	0
Salad dressing, fat-free, 1 tsp.	2	0	0	0	0

TABLE 5

Fat Grams in Dairy Foods

Food	Calories	Protein (g)	Total Fat (g)	Saturated Fat (g)	Cholesterol (mg)
Milk, whole, 1 cup	150	8	8	5	33
Milk, 2%, 1 cup	121	8	5	3	18
Milk, skim, 1 cup	86	8	0	0	4
Cheese, 1 oz.	114	7	9	4	30
Reduced-fat cheese, 1 oz.	71	8	5	3	10
Whole milk, plain yogurt, 8 oz.	139	8	7	5	29
Low-fat plain yogurt, 8 oz.	144	12	4	2	14
Fat-free, plain yogurt, 8 oz.	127	13	0	0	4

TABLE 6

Fat Grams in Non-Meat Protein Foods

Food	Calories	Protein (g)	Total Fat (g)	Saturated Fat (g)	Cholesterol (mg)
Black beans, 1/2 cup	109	7	0	0	0
Lentils, 1/2 cup	115	9	0	0	0
Garbanzo beans, 1/2 cup	143	6	1	0	0
Regular tofu, 6 oz.	104	11	6	1	0
Lite tofu, 6 oz.	71	12	2	0	0
Textured vegetable protein, 1/4 cup	58	11	0	0	0
Kidney beans, 1/2 cup	151	9	1	0	0

TABLE 7

Fat Grams in Meat Servings
*(Each 3-ounce serving of these meats, trimmed
of visible fat, provides 200 calories or less.)*

Cut of Meat	Calories	Protein (g)	Total Fat (g)	Saturated Fat (g)	Cholesterol (mg)
Pork tenderloin	159	26	5	2	80
Canadian bacon	157	21	7	2	49
Pork sirloin	181	24	9	3	72
Pork center loin	199	22	11	4	68
Whole ham	125	19	5	2	44
Beef tenderloin	179	24	8	3	71
Beef top sirloin	166	26	6	2	76
Beef sirloin strip steak	176	24	8	3	64
Beef top round	153	27	4	1	71
Beef round eye	149	25	5	2	59
Beef round tip sirloin roast	157	24	6	2	69
Beef flank steak	176	23	9	4	57
Veal leg	128	24	3	1	88
Lamb loin chop	184	25	8	3	81
Lamb foreshank	159	26	5	2	88
Lamb sirloin leg	173	24	8	3	78
Chicken breast, skinless	140	26	3	1	72
Chicken, dark meat, skinless	178	22	9	3	81
Turkey, light meat, skinless	119	26	1	0	73
Turkey, dark meat, skinless	159	24	6	2	72

TABLE 8
Fat Grams in Nuts and Seeds

Food	Calories	Protein (g)	Total Fat (g)	Saturated Fat (g)	Cholesterol (mg)
Soy nuts, 2 tbs.	48	4	3	0	0
Peanuts, 2 tbs.	104	5	9	1	0
Peanut butter, 2 tbs.	188	8	16	3	0
Chopped black walnuts, 2 tbs.	95	4	9	1	0
Almonds, 2 tbs.	101	3	9	1	0
Cashews, 2 tbs.	94	3	8	2	0
Pumpkin seeds, 2 tbs.	36	1	2	0	0
Sunflower seeds, 2 tbs.	93	3	8	1	0
Large dried brazilnuts, 5 ea.	155	3	16	4	0

TABLE 9
Fat Grams in Grain-Based Foods

Food	Calories	Protein (g)	Total Fat (g)	Saturated Fat (g)	Cholesterol (mg)
Whole wheat roll, 1	75	2	1	0	0
Croissant, 1	231	5	12	7	38
Potato chips, 1 oz.	152	2	10	3	0
Tortilla chips, 1 oz.	142	2	7	1	0
Plain bagel, 1	195	7	1	0	0
Tortilla, 1	159	4	3	1	0
Snack crackers, 6	90	1	5	1	0
Chocolate chip cookie, 1	78	1	5	1	5
Graham cracker, 1	29	0	1	0	0
Prepared pasta salad, 1/2 cup	187	11	8	2	3
Cooked pasta, 1/2 cup	99	3	0	0	0

The following foods have negligible fat grams:

Egg whites

Nonfat egg substitute

Nonfat cheese

Fruit (except coconuts and avocados)

Vegetables

Nonfat milk

Nonfat sour cream

Nonfat cream cheese

Nonfat yogurt

Fat-free margarine

Fat-free mayonnaise

Fat-free salad dressings

Keep in mind that these foods are not calorie free, and you'll have to accommodate their calorie content. You may choose to buy a calorie and fat counter to keep closer track of the nutritional content of your food choices.

Into the Kitchen: Two More Strategies

You're now well on the way to dieting success. Just to push you a little further toward your goals, we're going to help you with two more details: creating the low-fat pantry (ingredients you should have on hand that make food more enjoyable and interesting), and low-fat cooking techniques.

Creating the Low-Fat Pantry

Making interesting, lower-calorie food means turning up the flavor. Here are some pantry items that will help you get maximum flavor whenever possible.

Must haves:

Black peppercorns

Broth—chicken, beef, vegetable

Canned beans (white, kidney, garbanzo, lentils, black-eyed peas)

Capers

Cayenne pepper

Chinese five spice

Cocoa powder

Coconut milk, lite

Corn syrup

Cumin, ground

Curry powder

Dried fruits (apricots, prunes, dates, raisins, peaches, currants, cranberries, cherries)

Extracts (vanilla, rum, chocolate, coconut)

Flour—all purpose, cake, whole wheat, whole wheat pastry

Fruit butters (apple, peach, pineapple)

Fruit juices and nectars (papaya, apricot, pear, peach)

Garlic, fresh and powdered

Ginger, fresh and ground

Herbs, fresh and dried

Hoisin sauce

Honey

Jams and jellies, assorted fruit-juice-sweetened marmalades and chutneys

Ketchup

Kosher salt or sea salt

Maple syrup

Molasses

Mustards—Dijon, yellow, whole-grain

No-salt-added canned tomato products (paste, sauce, whole, crushed)

Nuts (pecans, walnuts)

Oils—canola, olive

Onion powder

Paprika, sweet Hungarian and hot

Peppers, dried

Pine nuts

Rice—brown, white, and also wild rice if you like it

Saffron (ask for it at customer service in your grocery or specialty foods store)

Sesame oil, dark (may be called roasted)

Soy sauce, reduced-sodium

Sun-dried tomatoes (not packed in oil)

Turmeric

Vegetable oil spray (plain and flavored)

Vinegar: balsamic, fruit-flavored, rice wine, white wine

Whole nutmeg

Worcestershire sauce, regular

Optional

Chili oil

Miso

Olives

Peppercorns, white or pink

Vinegar, red wine

Worcestershire sauce, white

Low-Fat Cooking Techniques:

- For cooking meat, fish, and poultry use one of the following techniques:

  Steam

  Stir "sizzle" (like stir-frying but use broth instead of oil)

  Roast

  Poach

  Braise

  Bake in parchment paper

- Toast or roast spices and nuts to intensify flavor. Do this by placing spices or nuts in a dry nonstick sauté pan and toss over medium heat for 3 or 4 minutes, until lightly toasted.
- Intensify the flavor of margarine or butter, so you can use less, by melting fresh herbs in it.
- Extend butter or margarine by mixing it with citrus juices or flavored vinegars.

- Use no-calorie flavoring extracts to replace high-calorie ingredients, such as coconut and rum extracts instead of the real thing.
- Replace high-fat ingredients with lower-fat alternatives. For example, use Canadian bacon or turkey bacon for regular bacon in recipes.
- Use smaller amounts of high-fat, high-calorie ingredients, but cut them up finely to disperse them throughout the food. For example, instead of coarsely chopped nuts, chop them finely; the same is true for olives. Another example: when a recipe calls for chocolate chips, use mini-morsels and cut the quantity in half.
- Use the most intensely flavored form of a food or ingredient. For example, choose extra-virgin olive oil over other types because it has the strongest flavor, and use Kosher or sea salt instead of regular table salt.
- Grease pans and muffin tins with vegetable oil spray instead of regular oil.
- Stir-fry with vegetable oil spray and broth instead of oil; alternatively, use very small amounts of an intensely flavored oil, such as dark sesame oil.
- Choose the leanest cuts of meat and use them consistently; inject variety by cutting the meat into different sizes and shapes.
- Use nonstick cookware and utensils so that you can use less fat.
- When making soups and stocks, always leave enough time to let them chill and then skim the fat off the top.
- Substitute reduced-fat and fat-free dairy products for regular varieties (milk, sour cream, cream cheese, yogurt, cheese). Experiment and determine when you can use each one and enjoy it; for example, sometimes nonfat cream cheese is acceptable in a recipe but not on a bagel. Similarly, reduced-fat cheese may melt on top of a casserole, but nonfat will not.
- Use strongly flavored cheeses such as feta and goat, but use much less of them.
- Marinate meats and vegetables in low-fat and fat-free marinades to intensify flavor.
- Replace fat flavor with sweet flavor. For example, use fruit salsas with pork, lamb, and fish; and marmalades with poultry.
- Use a food processor to help you chop, cut, and grate vegetables for recipes; you're more likely to prepare recipes containing these ingredients if you have some help.
- If you don't like to prepare fresh vegetables, buy frozen vegetables or fresh items in the produce section that are already cut into pieces. This can be a big help in getting more veggies into your diet.

The Real World: Eating Out

Eating out is one of the most difficult situations for any dieter to manage. Almost everyone tends to overeat when they eat out, even the non-dieters of the world. Here are some secrets that will help you enjoy eating out; after all, going out is supposed to be enjoyable, not stressful.

- Did you enter the restaurant ravenously hungry? Order a fruit cup as an appetizer.
- When you sit down, tell the server not to bring the dessert cart by your table after dinner. The beginning of the meal is when your resolve is highest.
- Don't see anything lean and light on the menu? Ask the server if the chef can broil a fish fillet or chicken breast.
- Do menus always tempt your taste buds beyond your willpower? Politely refuse the menu and order grilled fish or meat, a baked potato, steamed vegetables, and a salad with light dressing on the side.
- Order salads carefully and be suspicious of hidden fats; that healthy salad can become an instant fat landmine with the amount of dressing it's smothered in at most restaurants. Order dressing on the side and ask for a reduced-fat variety.
- Grilled burgers can get you into real trouble if the restaurant has buttered and grilled the bun (as they often do) or melted a huge hunk of cheese on it or smothered it in their secret sauce (a code word for butter, dressing, or some other high-fat item). Just ask the server for a dry bun and burger, maybe with some mustard or ketchup, and lots of lettuce and tomatoes.
- A sandwich of lean breast of turkey or some other healthy choice quickly becomes a fat nightmare if you forget to ask the deli to leave off the mayo and butter. They typically lather on several tablespoons of mayo, which breaks anyone's fat budget. Order your sandwich on dry bread, with mustard on the side, and fix it up yourself.
- Broiled fish can also be a fat fiasco for the unwary. Many restaurants add seasoned butter when they broil fish. Ask for it grilled and add your own lime or lemon juice.
- Ask for a plain baked potato and add your own sour cream or butter—but just a little. Alternatively, try lemon juice, salt, and pep-

per. You might even enjoy the great taste of the potato with nothing on it.

What If I'm Tempted to Eat a Very High-Fat Food?

You'll have to weigh this decision quite carefully. Certainly, you don't want to eat something such as a 40- to 50-gram-of-fat fast-food meal (which is easy to do with just a sandwich and fries, and sometimes with just a sandwich alone) while you are taking Xenical. The gastrointestinal consequences could be considerable. Here are possible options, with some solutions better then others:

- Wash away the desire. Drink a glass of water (or two or three); doing so has a cleansing action for the temptations of eating excessive fat grams.
- Figure out how much of the food you can eat and still stay within your limits. Remember, you probably only want a taste anyway. Enjoy a quarter of the hamburger and a handful of fries, then finish off your meal with a big salad. You'll be proud of yourself.
- Skip the Xenical and eat what you want. This isn't ideal at all; it sets a dangerous precedent. But if the options are gastrointestinal discomfort or absorbing all the fat grams you eat, you will have to make the choice. If you take this route more than a couple of times, then you need to ask yourself if you are really a candidate for the Xenical plan.

This concludes the diet portion of the Xenical program. Now let's see the incredible benefits exercise can bring to your weight and health.

c h a p t e r

6

Exercising with Xenical: Designing Your Individual Fat-Burning Program

You're two-thirds of the way toward achieving a slimmer life you will enjoy and relish long into your golden years. You've learned how to modify your eating plans for better health, and you're taking Xenical to give you the dieting advantage.

But you're still missing one crucial step: exercise. Research couldn't be more clear that exercising consistently is one of the key strategies in living a healthier life. Indeed, scientists have demonstrated that people who incorporate regular exercise into their lives are more successful at shedding excess pounds, as well as keeping them off long-term, than those who don't exercise regularly. I have seen this firsthand over and over again.

"I don't have time."

"It will ruin my hair."

"I don't know how to exercise."

"I don't have any exercise equipment."

These are all excuses I have heard over the many years I have been helping men and women lose weight. The list of reasons TO exercise is even longer, though; it is so much more than just burning calories. We've divided these reasons into two categories: why exercise is so crucial to weight loss, and the myriad other reasons to stay active. Let's start with the reasons that exercise is so crucial to weight-loss success:

- Exercise speeds up metabolism, the rate at which the body burns calories. Chronic dieting, the so-called yo-yo dieting, slows metabolism—in a separate way from the body's calorie-conserving starvation strategy that we discussed on pages 47–48. In fact, there's nothing magical about the way repeated weight loss and regain affects this aspect of metabolism at all. Actually, it's the type of weight people lose and then the type they regain that is so devastating to metabolism. Let me explain. Most people lose some muscle mass, in addition to fat, when they lose weight, especially if they diet by cutting calories and not exercising. But most people who regain weight after losing tend to regain more fat than muscle. With each cycle of loss and gain, the percentage of body muscle mass decreases and the percentage of fat increases, which slows metabolism more and more. However, when you include exercise in your weight-loss plan from the start, you prevent this loss of precious muscle, saving yourself the job of building it back. Let's turn preserving muscle mass into numbers you can get excited about. Every day, each pound of muscle burns 35 to 50 calories (even at rest), compared to a measly 2 calories for each pound of fat. Over time a few—or even one—extra pound of muscle can help keep the pounds from piling back on. Even while you sleep, muscle tissue burns at least seventeen times as many calories as fat tissue.
- Exercise helps prevent the body from turning its metabolism down to a starvation-conservation mode. Remember that amazing survival mechanism I told you about earlier? It happens when the body thinks the food supply is dangerously low and so jumps back to the ancient survival skill of operating on fewer calories. Fortunately, exercise can break this cycle, but it is also important not to cut calories too dramatically.

The non-weight-loss benefits of exercise are so many and so great that it is not possible to list them all here. Here are just a few:

- Exercise lowers blood pressure. In fact, it may be one of the most effective nondrug therapies for lowering blood pressure. When researchers studied the effects of walking in people with normal blood pressure, they found that a regular program of walking lowered systolic blood pressure (that's the top number) by 6 to 8 mm Hg (millimeters of mercury, the unit by which blood pressure is measured) and diastolic pressure (the bottom number) by 7 mm Hg.
- Regular exercise lowers heart attack risk. A Finnish study involving

nearly fifteen hundred men revealed that those who exercised regularly slashed their risk of heart attack by about one-third. In fact, lack of exercise in and of itself is a separate risk factor for having a heart attack.

- Exercise raises HDL cholesterol, the good cholesterol that helps clear bad cholesterol from the bloodstream.
- Stepping up your pace increases functional capacity, or the ability of the heart to use oxygen more efficiently. In the long run, this means that each physical effort requires less work from the heart.
- Staying active helps prevent the onset and progression of type 2, or non-insulin-dependent diabetes, often called adult-onset diabetes.
- Regularly working up a sweat holds disability, disease, and even death at bay, according to an eight-year study of approximately eight hundred middle-aged and older adults. Study participants who frequently engaged in some form of vigorous physical activity had lower blood pressure, took fewer medications, visited their doctors less frequently, and were less likely to die prematurely.
- Exercise is a great stress reducer. Reducing stress helps you better manage day-to-day upsets, work more efficiently, and look at life's cup as half full rather than as half empty. Come to think of it, we could even put this reason for exercising in the previous listing because some people eat out of stress, and often indiscriminately so. Perhaps you've even done it yourself—stopped at the bakery or vending machine after a particularly harrowing day, hoping that a doughnut or candy bar would ease the stress. Usually, though, eating this way just adds to your stress level. So change to a tried and true way to eliminate stress and stress-related eating: exercise.
- Exercise improves self-concept, mood, and even the ability to think clearly. This reason, too, could be placed in the list of reasons to exercise for weight-loss purposes. Putting a positive spin on your self-concept is an exceptionally effective way to give yourself the encouragement you need to keep up the effort to lose weight.

About Our Exercise Program

We've taken the guesswork out of exercising, guiding you every step of the way. For starters, we walk you through the pre-exercise planning stage, which is so very important to exercising safely. We give you some information on selecting an exercise program you can stick with for life. In addition, we've thoroughly addressed how long and how vigorously you should exercise.

If you have never exercised—or if it has been a long time since you have—don't worry. Our very basic walking program, Exercise Program Number One, is great for everyone, even those who might be concerned about stepping out their front door with their sneakers on for the first time. And for those of you who have been engaging in regular physical activity, we've provided a more challenging cross-training program that should keep exercise interesting for you.

We've also made no bones about the importance of weight training, or weight lifting as some people call it. It is a great aid to long-term weight loss and weight maintenance, to say nothing of living healthier and more independently into your golden years. We've provided lots of guidance to get you going on an easy program of weight training.

To help you keep track of your increasing fitness level, we've included forms for you to photocopy and use to chart your progress. And that's key to success. Now let's get moving.

Before You Start

Consult your physician. The importance of exercise to good health is nearly immeasurable, but so is the medical checkup you need before you embark on any new program. Let's say, for example, that you have been enjoying a casual walk every day after dinner for ten or fifteen minutes (congratulations, by the way, because that is a great start!). Let's say you now want to start playing racquetball two nights per week and jog another couple of nights, both of which will help you increase your calorie expenditure.

As you can imagine, there is a big difference in these two levels of exercise. Just to make sure you and your heart are ready to embark on more strenuous exercise, make it a top priority to talk about your planned routine with your physician when you are discussing using Xenical. Based on your medical history and age, your physician will know what kinds of tests to run to determine your exercise capacity. The information your physician gathers is key to designing an exercise program that will help rather than hurt you.

Start slowly. Starting slowly and gradually increasing your strength and endurance is critical to your persevering over the long haul. If you start out at full force, you may pull a muscle or wind up so sore that you won't continue after a day or two. Also, you may be so fatigued that you can't imagine keeping up such a pace for the rest of your life.

Choose Critically: Love How You Move

Make It Livable for Life. Yes, hammering away on the stair climber for an hour is a great way to burn calories, as is running for an hour daily. But ask yourself if the exercise you've chosen is one you want to do long-term. Just as you need to commit to the dietary changes you're making while on Xenical, you need to make sure that the exercise plan you choose is easily incorporated it into your daily lifestyle. Otherwise, you just won't stay with it.

Go for Variety. Over the years I have learned from my patients—as well as from my own exercise life—that trying lots of different types of exercise may be the best plan of all. We call this cross-training. For example, enjoy a brisk walk one day, a vigorous swim another, and a spin on your bicycle another day. Incorporate golf, tennis, volleyball, and other fun activities on a regular basis. You'll find that exercise is no longer a chore but one of the most enjoyable aspects of your life.

Adding variety to your exercise routine, or cross-training, has some great advantages. First, it strengthens more muscle groups. In terms of weight loss, that means revving up the calorie-burning capacity of more muscles in your body, or increasing your metabolic rate. And there are two other advantages: You're less likely to become bored with exercise; therefore you're more likely to continue exercising over a longer period of time. You're also less likely to suffer an overuse injury, which can keep you from exercising and burning calories.

Should I Buy Exercise Equipment? It's almost impossible to sort through all the types of equipment, or even the many models of one particular type of equipment in the average sporting goods store. But do you actually need exercise equipment? Only if you want a particular item. Although most equipment has some benefit, there's no reason to go out and buy it if you haven't been exercising. It is better to start with a walking program or perhaps a swimming program to determine what you like to do when it comes to exercise. In other words, don't spend money on equipment hoping it will change your lifestyle. Change your lifestyle and then carefully consider what equipment might enhance your exercise routine.

How Much You Should Exercise

For health reasons alone—to strengthen the heart and lungs, for example—the latest research indicates that everyone should exercise at moderate intensity a minimum of thirty minutes most days of the week. This advice stems from the 1995 National Institutes of Health Consensus Development Conference Statement on Physical Activity and Cardiovascular Health. Moderate-intensity exercise is commonly called aerobic exercise.

Put another way, burning as few as 1,000 calories weekly in exercise is enough to improve health and lower heart attack and stroke risk, according to heart experts. How much exercise is that? It translates into walking at about 2½ to 3 miles per hour for thirty minutes about five days per week. One trick that exercise experts allow to help you get the heart benefits quickly: if you're short on time, you can exercise at a higher intensity for twenty minutes to give your heart the workout it needs.

The good news is that if you don't have time for a thirty-minute brisk walk, you can divide the thirty minutes into several smaller sessions. For example, you can park your car a brisk ten-minute walk away from the office. Making that trip twice daily will wipe out twenty of the thirty minutes. To get the other ten minutes, jump on your exercise bike or grab the dog for a quick constitutional after dinner. It's not as hard as it seems!

If you're just starting to exercise, begin with shorter bursts of activity, say fifteen to twenty minutes of exercise every other day. Progress slowly, by three- to five-minute increments per week, until you are at your exercise goal: thirty minutes most (and preferably all) days of the week.

Finally, note that prolonging your exercise sessions might help you burn more calories over the long haul, although not all weight-loss experts agree on this point. Ideally, we'd like to find a way to help you increase your metabolism for hours, not just during the time you are exercising. There is some evidence that exercising vigorously for at least forty-five minutes at each session may help accomplish this. You can reap the same benefits for your heart and lungs by exercising in shorter bursts, but you may give yourself the weight-loss advantage by sweating through a routine for at least forty-five minutes. This might be especially true if you exercise at higher rather than lower intensities. In the long run, this extra activity may prolong your increased calorie-burning power even after you've stopped exercising.

How Vigorously You Should Exercise

Moderate-intensity exercise, or aerobic exercise, is the recommended activity level. Aerobic exercise should cause you to break a sweat, breathe more heavily than usual, and use the large muscle groups of the body. Examples include brisk walking, swimming, jogging, dancing, and hiking. More strenuous exercise, such as stair climbing or running, is fine but not necessary to reap health benefits.

Exercising at moderate intensity translates into working at 60 to 70 percent of your maximum heart rate. Your maximum heart rate is approximately 220 minus your age, so you can calculate your target heart rate range for exercise by taking 60 to 70 percent of this value. For example, if you are forty, here's how to calculate your target heart rate:

Step 1: 220 − 40 = 180 beats per minute

Step 2: 180 × .60 = 108 beats per minute

Step 3: 180 × .70 = 126 beats per minute

Target heart rate = 108 to 126 beats per minute

As an alternative to checking your heart rate, just be sure to exercise at an intensity that causes you to breathe more heavily than usual but at which you can still carry on a conversation.

If you have not been exercising, start slowly—aiming for a heart rate lower than your target heart rate—to avoid muscle injury and over-taxing your heart and lungs, which are accustomed to a more sedentary lifestyle. (See the next section, "How Vigorously You Should Exercise," to learn how to calculate your target heart rate.) No matter how great your motivation to engage in aerobic exercise, your heart and lungs cannot meet the demand immediately. Your cardiovascular system and muscles also perform better and are less likely to suffer negative effects when you include a five- to fifteen-minute warm-up and cool-down period.

Concentrate and Squeeze More Calories Out of Your Workout

Take advantage of the mind-body connection to exercise at a higher intensity and burn more calories, say exercise experts. It all boils down to a strategy used by athletes, who learn to "associate" with their bodies and "dissociate" from the rest of the world during workouts. That means they pay attention to what each muscle and part of their body is doing and how it is performing. At the same time, they tune out extraneous environmental noise, using extra powers of concentration to push their muscles to perform harder. Runners, for example, concentrate on pumping their arms harder and increasing their stride as well as the power behind each stride. What does this mean for you? Turn off the television and instead find music that tends to jazz up your exercise routine. Concentrate on the muscles that are working and drive them a little further each time with that mind-body connection.

Top Ten Fat-Burning Exercises

Clearly, it's better to choose an activity you look forward to doing. Hate the exercise bike? We give you permission never to get on it. Love vacuuming? Then find every last piece of dust and lint under the beds, couches, and in the closets every day. If you're versatile and are truly searching for maximum calorie-burning exercises, consult our list below for the activity that burns up the most calories.* Just make sure you enjoy whatever you choose, or you'll find your way back to couch-potato status in a big hurry.

Activity	Calories Burned per 30 Minutes
Biking, 15 mph (fairly fast)	188
Biking, 10 mph (more leisurely)	171
Gardening (heavy, such as mowing and digging)	214
Golf (walk with bag)	202
Housework (heavy)	202
Jogging (10-minute miles)	295
Swimming (moderately fast)	173
Tennis (moderate)	188
Walking, 3 mph (moderate)	95
Walking, 5 mph (fast)	226

* Calories are for a 150-pound person; a lighter-weight person will burn fewer calories per hour, while a heavier person will burn more.

Exercise Program Number One: Walking

Here is a great starting exercise program for someone who has not been exercising and is feeling out of shape. Photocopy the chart at the end of this section and use it to follow your progress.

Before you step out the door or onto the treadmill, stretch your leg muscles. Stand with both hands against the wall, not quite an arm's length away from the wall. Place one foot close to the wall and the other about two feet away from the wall. You should be standing on the ball of the foot that is behind you. Stretch the heel of this foot down toward the ground slowly and hold for a count of twenty. Reverse feet and repeat. Now you are ready to hit the road.

Monday

- Start walking at a slow, leisurely pace. You will notice no increase in heart rate and will not break a sweat. Continue for five to ten minutes.
- For the next fifteen minutes, step up the pace just to where you notice the difference; you should perspire and your heart rate should increase.
- Stroll leisurely again for five to ten minutes.

Tuesday

Rest.

Wednesday

- Start walking at a slow, leisurely pace, with no increase in heart rate and not breaking a sweat. Continue for five to ten minutes.
- For the next fifteen minutes, step up the pace just to where you notice the difference; you should perspire and your heart rate should increase.
- Stroll leisurely again for five to ten minutes.

Thursday

Rest.

Friday

- Start walking at a slow, leisurely pace, with no increase in heart rate and not breaking a sweat. Continue for five to ten minutes.
- For the next seventeen minutes, step up the pace just to where you notice the difference; you should perspire and your heart rate should increase.
- Stroll leisurely again for five to ten minutes.

Saturday

- Start walking at a faster pace, where you notice a slight increase in heart rate and break a slight sweat. Continue for five to ten minutes.
- For the next seventeen minutes, step up the pace just to where you notice the difference; you should perspire and your heart rate should increase, and you should travel a little farther than you did on Friday.
- Stroll leisurely again for five to ten minutes.

Sunday

Rest.

During the second week exercise an extra day, working out on days 1, 3, 4, 6, and 7. Also increase the aerobic portion of your workout to twenty minutes on days 6 and 7.

During the third week, participate in your walking routine on days 1, 2, 3, 5, 6, 7, striving for twenty aerobic minutes each day.

During the fourth week add the seventh day and increase your distance during the twenty minutes.

Congratulations! You are well on the way to being fit. You have established a healthy exercise pattern that you can adhere to for life. Where you go from here is up to you. You can continue to step up the pace during the aerobic portion of your workout, or you can increase the time for this portion. You need only a half hour of exercise to have a fit heart and lungs, but exercising more can help you lose more pounds and also keep them off. Another option is to move on to other forms of exercise, which we call cross-training. Finally, you can choose to walk every day during some weeks, and cross-train during other weeks. The possibilities are endless—and trying lots of different activities should keep you interested and motivated.

My Walking Program

Week Number _____

Day of the Week	Minutes of Warm-Up	Minutes of Walking	Distance Walked
Monday			
Tuesday			
Wednesday			
Thursday			
Friday			
Saturday			
Sunday			

Exercise Program Number Two: Cross-Training

Try this plan if you want more variety in your workout. If some of the exercises don't work for you, then substitute another that you enjoy more. Just don't cut back on the time we've indicated. Photocopy the chart following the program, write in the exercise you choose for each day, and indicate how many minutes you enjoy it.

Week	Monday	Tuesday	Wednesday	Thursday	Friday	Saturday	Sunday
1	30 minutes walking	30 minutes tennis	30 minutes yard raking	30 minutes exercise bike	rest	30 minutes walking	30 minutes minutes washing floors
2	rest	30 minutes walking	30 minutes tennis	30 minutes vacuuming	30 minutes swimming	30 minutes walking	30 minutes exercise bike
3	30 minutes walking	rest	30 minutes swimming	30 minutes volleyball	30 minutes walking	30 minutes vacuuming	30 minutes tennis
4	rest	30 minutes jogging	30 minutes exercise bike	30 minutes walking	30 minutes washing floors	30 minutes exercise bike	30 minutes tennis
5	30 minutes walking	rest	30 minutes swimming	30 minutes vacuuming	30 minutes walking	30 minutes bicycling	30 minutes volleyball

Chart Your Own Progress in Cross-Training

Monday	Tuesday	Wednesday	Thursday	Friday	Saturday	Sunday

Weight Training: Help Your Body Help You Lose Weight

Forty-eight-year-old Mary, a corporate recruiter in Cleveland, Ohio, has to maximize every moment of her time, and that includes the few she has left for staying healthfully trim. "I used to have to spend a great amount of time on aerobic workouts every day and still fight to maintain my ideal body weight," said Mary, who added that she was always hungry because she tried to eat less after age forty to avoid the "middle-age spread." "Once I started weight training, I found I had to work out less to stay in shape and not gain weight."

Eight years into her exercise routine, Mary hasn't faltered from her three-times-per-week weight-training routine and is thrilled with the results. She did more than stop the creeping pounds: she has toned up and dropped a clothing size. "I'm nearly fifty but am still pleased with how I look in sleeveless shirts and shorts," says Mary proudly.

Mary discovered that weight training adds muscle—fighting the trend of muscle loss due to aging. As a normal consequence of each passing year, adult bodies want to give up muscle mass. This is especially true in areas of the body that even regular aerobic exercisers such as bikers, walkers, and joggers don't work out—the upper body. No matter how much you work out aerobically, your body still needs weight training.

So why didn't our forefathers have to hoist dumbbells to stay Tarzan sleek? Actually, they did pump iron, just in a different way. Most of the tasks for which we now push a button once required a whole lot more sweat and aching muscles—right down to licking an envelope and walking a letter to the mailbox. For many of us even that has been simplified to an e-mail click. If you think about it, some people could lie in bed and maintain their career, given a phone, modem, and laptop computer.

How much time does it take Mary—or, for that matter, anyone—to weight-train? Not as much as you'd think. She follows the guidelines of the American College of Sports Medicine (ACSM), which recommends performing eight to ten different exercises in two to three weight training sessions weekly. Choose a range of exercises that improve strength in all the major muscle groups, especially those that help you do everyday activities such as lifting a bag of groceries or starting the lawnmower. This becomes especially important as we age, when something as simple as pouring milk from a gallon container can become difficult for people who don't maintain muscular strength.

Remember that muscles will be maintained only if you challenge them, so modify or intensify your routine as necessary. Choosing the correct weight is essential to strengthening muscles without injuring them. Start with a weight that causes muscle fatigue after one set of about eight to twelve repetitions. In other words, if you can lift the weight thirteen to fifteen times, it probably isn't heavy enough, but if you can't hoist it at least eight times, then it's too heavy. For some exercises you may need three pounds, and for others as much as fifteen.

One set of repetitions is plenty, says ACSM. Older guidelines recommended more than one set of repetitions, but continuing research found little benefit in that—and people were less likely to continue weight training for a long time when faced with such guidelines. Rest at least two days before working a muscle group again. Injuries are far more common in people who overzealously weight-train the same muscle groups two days in a row.

How soon will it be before you see results? Most people see significant results—a trimmer, more toned physique—within eight weeks. Remember that even while you are resting, each pound of muscle burns 35 to 50 calories per day. Compare that to a measly 2 calories burned by each pound of fat. A body with more muscles burns more calories all day long. It's no wonder that the classic research studies found that after only twelve weeks, participants in a regular program of weight training increased their calorie needs by 15 percent. This means that if they are not eating any more calories, their weight loss will be speedier as a result of their weight training.

Here are some more guidelines about weight training:
• Don't worry about bulking up or gaining too much muscle mass. It's almost impossible to do so unless you lift excessive weights for a long period of time. Done properly, weight training transforms your body into a firm, sleek specimen—and one that burns fuel faster.

- You don't have to buy expensive weight-lifting equipment—even soup cans or bags of rice will do. Plastic milk containers will also work; if they are too heavy when they are full, wait until they are empty and then fill with varying levels of sand. If you are buying equipment, it is better to buy weights of varying sizes than a bar with weight plates. This is because people often misuse the bar with weight plates. To avoid the time and frustration of adding and removing plates on such bars, people tend to use the same weight for all exercises, which either doesn't challenge some muscles or injures others.

Basic Weight-Training Exercises

The two sets of exercises given below are for two different sets of muscles. Each exercise should be repeated ten to fifteen times. It is important that you keep these exercises divided into the groups we have put them in, to avoid injury. You can become injured if you exercise the same muscle groups two days in a row. If you have any doubt about how to perform these exercises, don't do them. Instead, seek help from a local fitness club or Y. Finally, make copies of our charts and use them to keep track of your progress.

Monday, Wednesday, and Friday Weight-Training Exercises

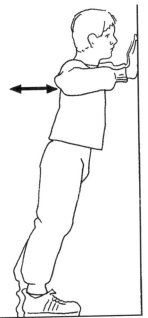

Wall push-up: Stand about 2½ feet from a wall. Place hands on the wall at shoulder height. Lower yourself slowly toward the wall, then push your body away from it.

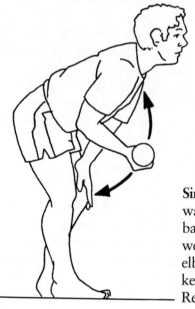

Single arm row: Bend forward from the waist. Rest left hand on knee, keeping back flat and knees slightly bent. Start with weight in right hand, arm extended and elbow unlocked. Pull weight to shoulder, keeping arm close to body. Lower weight. Repeat on other side.

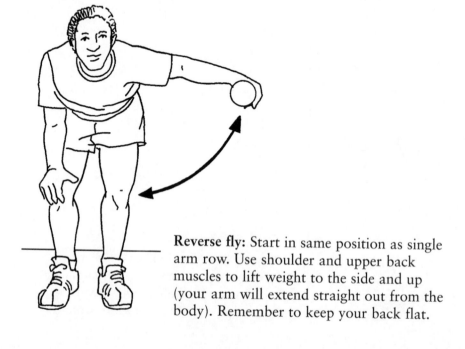

Reverse fly: Start in same position as single arm row. Use shoulder and upper back muscles to lift weight to the side and up (your arm will extend straight out from the body). Remember to keep your back flat.

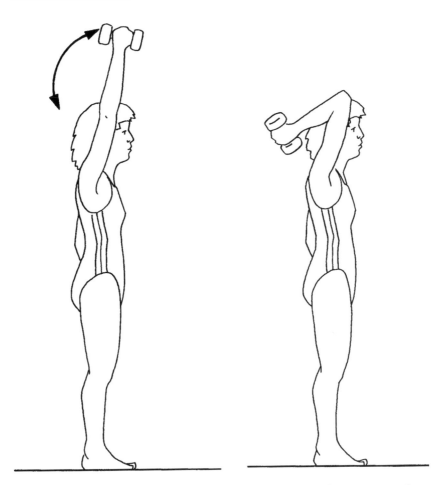

Tricep press: Start with weight above head, palm facing inward. Lower weight to your back, then raise to starting position. Support elbow with opposite hand if necessary, keeping arm close to head.

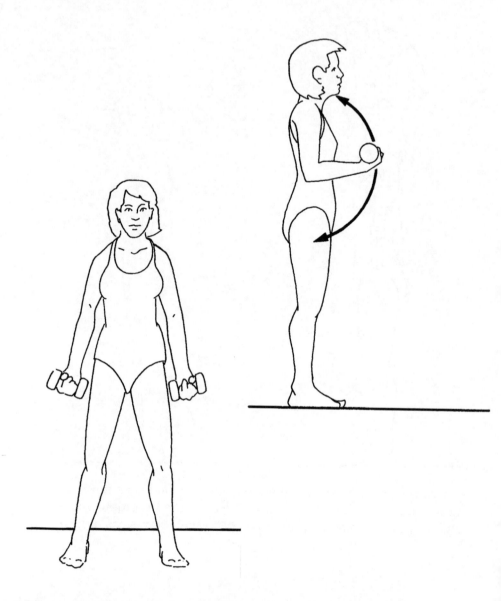

Bicep curl: Stand with feet shoulder width apart, arms by sides. Hold weights in hands, palms facing forward. Keeping elbows close to sides, raise weights to chin level, then lower.

Chart Your Progress

MONDAY, WEDNESDAY, AND FRIDAY

Exercise	Weight Used			Number of Repetitions
	Mon.	Wed.	Fri.	
Wall Push-up				
Week One				
Week Two				
Week Three				
Week Four				
Week Five				
Week Six				
Single Arm Row				
Week One				
Week Two				
Week Three				
Week Four				
Week Five				
Week Six				
Reverse Fly				
Week One				
Week Two				
Week Three				
Week Four				
Week Five				
Week Six				
Tricep Press				
Week One				
Week Two				
Week Three				
Week Four				
Week Five				
Week Six				
Bicep Curl				
Week One				
Week Two				
Week Three				
Week Four				
Week Five				
Week Six				

Tuesday, Thursday, and Saturday Exercises

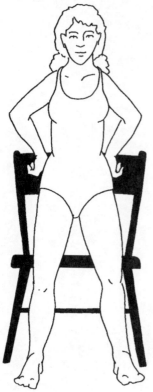

Chair squat: Stand with chair behind you, feet a little more than shoulder width apart. Lower yourself into the chair as if you are going to sit. Stand back up just before you actually sit. Keep back straight and put hands on hips or out in front of you as needed for balance.

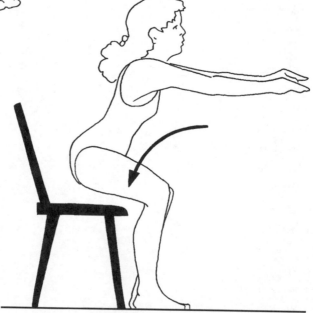

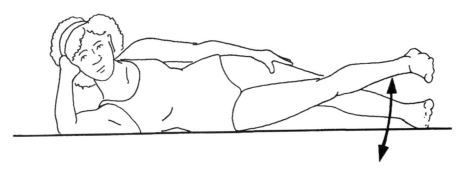

Inner thigh lift: Lie on side, hips, shoulders, and feet in straight line. Rest head on hand. Extend straight bottom leg forward and lift toward ceiling. Lower. Switch sides after set.

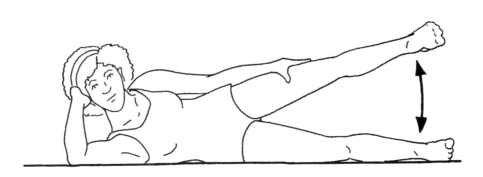

Outer thigh lift: Start in same position as inner thigh lift. Slowly lift and lower straight upper leg. Switch sides after set.

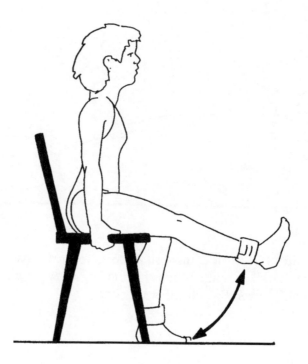

Seated lower leg lift: Sit on chair with back straight, feet flat on floor, hands grasping sides of chair for balance. Straighten leg, then lower foot back to floor. Do not lock knee. Start without using any weights, then add ankle weights as your muscles grow stronger.

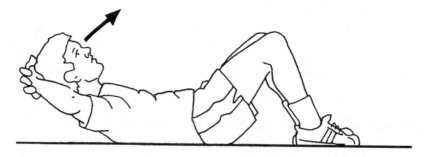

Abdominal crunches: Lie on the floor, knees bent, feet shoulder width apart. Place hands behind head. Keep elbows out, chin off chest. Raise head and shoulders off the floor. Lower back. Don't let head rest on floor in between reps. Don't pull your head up with your hands. Concentrate on pressing your belly button into the floor.

Chart Your Progress

TUESDAY, THURSDAY, SATURDAY

Exercise	Weight Used			Number of Repetitions
	Tues.	Thurs.	Sat.	
Chair Squat				
Week One				
Week Two				
Week Three				
Week Four				
Week Five				
Week Six				
Inner Thigh Lift				
Week One				
Week Two				
Week Three				
Week Four				
Week Five				
Week Six				
Outer Thigh Lift				
Week One				
Week Two				
Week Three				
Week Four				
Week Five				
Week Six				
Seated Lower Leg Lift				
Week One				
Week Two				
Week Three				
Week Four				
Week Five				
Week Six				
Abdominal Crunch				
Week One				
Week Two				
Week Three				
Week Four				
Week Five				
Week Six				

The Exercise Advantage

The most important thing is to get moving today—even if it means setting out on a five-minute stroll out your front door. That's a great start for someone who otherwise would have spent the time watching television. Then you're moving your body, getting the blood flowing and the calories burning. Set a goal of engaging in some form of physical activity almost every day, and settle for no less than six days each week. You may have more success at accomplishing your exercise goal if you try to exercise at the same time each day. In other words, try to set a routine.

Finally, as you close this chapter, do one more thing for yourself: link forever in your mind the words "exercise" and "diet." Now that you've given yourself the Xenical advantage in dieting, give yourself the exercise advantage, too. As I hope I've made clear, you increase immeasurably your success in losing weight when you step up your pace.

7

I've Hit My Goal Weight! Now What?

Congratulations! You've achieved a healthier weight that will help you live a longer, more vibrant life and reduce your risks from a host of dangerous diseases. You have every right to take pride in your appearance and all the hard work, self-control, and self-confidence it represents.

You're probably asking "Now what?" That certainly is a fair question. We are still here for you, to help you through this important transition period. Learning how to lose weight was difficult, but learning how to keep it off is just as difficult. Let's get started on this important lifelong task.

Before we do, though, I would like to remind you of one very important attitude that I try to instill in all my patients seeking weight loss, even before I help them start on a weight-loss strategy. Weight loss and weight maintenance are on a continuum. They are one way of life, not two separate lifestyles. The weight-loss lifestyle you have learned from this book now becomes the weight-maintenance lifestyle you will adhere to for life. Only small details change. To be specific, you'll stay with the healthy eating style you have learned and just vary the serving sizes and therefore the calories. (There are a couple of very minor changes to be discussed later.)

It is very frustrating to hear patients talk about dieting as if it were a temporary situation. Indeed, when people regard a weight-loss diet as an interim eating style, they invariably slip back to the way of eating that brought them to such an unhealthy weight. There is no such thing as dieting and not dieting, at least when it comes to success. Instead, there is a new way of life into which you have incorporated healthy eating, regular exercise, and a new self-respect that allows you to successfully make the changes you need for life.

Should You Keep Taking Xenical?

Once you have achieved your goal weight, you may choose to continue taking Xenical as you adjust to your weight-maintenance lifestyle. Our research indicates that this may help you keep the weight off. According to the Xenical research study I was involved in, those dieters who continued taking Xenical during the second year of the study, while following a weight maintenance diet, had an easier time keeping the weight off.

Do you remember my patient Cindy, the one who lost so much weight (and has kept it off for over four years)? She got her start on Xenical and then, after stopping the drug, continued to lose weight on her own. She also kept the weight off without the drug. I would say that Cindy is the ideal Xenical patient, representing the manner in which Xenical should be used. First, Cindy got the help she needed with Xenical to start losing weight. Second, after learning the Xenical way of dieting and exercise, Cindy was able to stop the drug and continue losing weight on her own. Last, Cindy learned how to change her lifestyle permanently, which allowed her to keep the weight off without having to take the drug.

When I asked Cindy what finally clicked for her—she had tried so many different dieting strategies before taking Xenical—she said, "I truly had to learn how to eat right with Xenical. There simply was no room for crash dieting or for bingeing." She added, "Xenical taught me how to live right and then gave me the confidence to do it on my own."

The best advice I can give you is to discuss with your physician your options for continuing Xenical after you have met your weight-loss goal. Remember, the big advantage to the Xenical diet and exercise program is that you have learned to modify your life overall, which makes living the slimmer life much easier once you stop taking the drug. This is because for Xenical to work properly you had to learn to eat low-fat meals consistently and also to enjoy very low-fat snacks. You wouldn't have reached this point of success if you hadn't done so.

The Weight-Maintenance Diet

The only difference between the Xenical weight-loss plan and the Xenical weight-maintenance diet is the calorie level. Although you lost weight on somewhere between 1,300 and 1,700 calories daily, you can now increase calories to somewhere between 1,800 and 2,000. The same healthy foods will be a part of your life forever. I am confident that you won't slip back into the old ways of eating that caused your original weight gain.

How do you decide how many more calories you can eat without gaining weight? I suggest that you experiment and increase calories slowly. If you've lost weight on 1,500 calories, for example, try increasing calories to 1,800 at first. If you lose weight on that over a month, then try moving up to 2,000. Our weight-maintenance plans include two calorie levels so that you can experiment along these lines. Just remember that very subtle changes in serving size make the difference between these calorie levels and that you must pay careful attention to serving size to be successful at weight maintenance.

Please note that Week One of our weight-maintenance menus are designed to accommodate the continued use of Xenical; that means you still need to restrict fat grams to a maximum of 20 per meal in order to minimize any side effects. If you decide to stop taking Xenical, however, you have a little more leeway on how to divide up your fat grams throughout the day. Week Two incorporates this flexibility, with some of the meals containing more than 20 grams of fat—although not much more throughout. This is because we want you to continue eating the Xenical way since it is the healthiest way you can eat. We always adhere to the 30 percent guidelines, never exceeding 30 percent of a day's calorie total as fat calories.

The other rules we have used in creating the weight-maintenance menus are as follows:

- Snacks are included. The body has an easier time burning smaller bundles of energy than larger ones, so including snacks and having slightly smaller meals become a very important way of life *for life.*
- Snacks are always low in fat. You learned this way of eating for a reason—because it is the healthiest way to eat—and we want you to continue it. Snacking on fruits, vegetables, fat-free dairy foods, and whole-grain cereal products is what health officials throughout the country recommend (whether or not you are trying to lose weight).

• The fiber content continues at the recommended healthy, high levels (at least 25 grams per day). Fiber is important to good health and helps you have a healthier intestinal tract; it reduces cholesterol levels and fights the tendency toward type 2 diabetes. Fiber also helps fill you up, satisfying your hunger with fewer calories (higher fiber foods are naturally lower in calories). Fiber may help you corral and get rid of some of the dietary fat you eat, according to the latest research.

Do you need a vitamin/mineral supplement now that you aren't losing weight? If you're not taking Xenical, the answer is probably no. We know that people who eat at least 1,800 calories a day generally can get all the nutrients their bodies need from their diet. You will be eating an exceptionally healthy diet for life, so I am confident that you are getting all essential vitamins and minerals. Health officials agree, saying that it is not necessary to take a supplement but it is much better to focus on eating healthfully and "harvesting" all nutrients from food.

> One exception might be an iron supplement for women who are still menstruating. It can be hard to get enough iron during these years, particularly if you are cutting down on red meat. The other exception might be calcium, and that may apply to men and women. Ask your physician if you need a calcium supplement.

The Xenical Weight-Maintenance Program

	WEEK ONE: FOR THOSE WHO CONTINUE TO TAKE XENICAL	
	Week One, Day One	
Food	1,800 calories	2,000 calories
BREAKFAST		
Broccoli , Mushroom, and Cheese Omelet	Recipe as shown	Recipe as shown
Whole wheat toast	1 slice	1 slice
Tub margarine	2 teaspoons	2 teaspoons
Skim milk	1 cup	1 cup
MORNING SNACK		
Grapenuts fruit salad: ¹/₂ cup blueberries sprinkled with ¹/₂ cup Grapenuts	1 serving	1 serving
LUNCH		
Tossed Shrimp Salad	Recipe as shown	Recipe as shown
Buttery round crackers (such as Ritz)	5	10
Skim milk	¹/₂ cup	1 cup
Fresh peach	1	1
AFTERNOON SNACK		
Whole-grain toast	1 slice	1 slice
Strawberry jam	1 teaspoon	1 teaspoon
Skim milk	¹/₂ cup	¹/₂ cup
DINNER		
Buttered Rotini with Chicken Stir-Fry	Recipe as shown	Recipe as shown
Skim milk	Omit	1 cup
Totally Decadent Banana Chocolate Chip Muffin	1	1

Week One, Day One (continued)

Food	1,800 calories	2,000 calories
EVENING SNACK		
Graham crackers	2	2
Nonfat cream cheese	1 tablespoon	1 tablespoon
NUTRITION TOTALS FOR DAY ONE		
Calories	1,813	2,026
Fat (g)	46	51
Carbohydrate (g)	266	295
Protein (g)	93	106
Fiber (g)	27	27
Calories from fat (%)	22	22

Week One, Day Two

Food	1,800 calories	2,000 calories
BREAKFAST		
Poached egg	1	2
Whole wheat toast	2 slices	2 slices
Tub margarine	2 teaspoons	2 teaspoons
Skim milk	1 cup	1 cup
MORNING SNACK		
Cantaloupe pieces	1 cup	2 cups
Vegetable juice cocktail	1 cup	1 cup
LUNCH		
Favorite Tuna Pasta Salad	¼ recipe	¼ recipe
Whole-grain rye crisp	5	5
Skim milk	1 cup	1 cup
AFTERNOON SNACK		
Fresh peach, sliced, with 1 teaspoon brown sugar	1 serving	1 serving
Skim milk	1 cup	1 cup

Food	1,800 calories	2,000 calories
DINNER		
Grilled salmon	5 ounces	5 ounces
Medium sweet potato, baked	1	1
Margarine	2 teaspoons	2 teaspoons
Broccoli, steamed	1 cup	1 cup
EVENING SNACK		
Nonfat frozen yogurt, favorite flavor	1 cup	1 1/2 cups
NUTRITION TOTALS FOR DAY TWO		
Calories	1,717	1,952
Fat (g)	40	47
Carbohydrate (g)	221	256
Protein (g)	131	144
Fiber (g)	25	27
Calories from fat (%)	21	21

Week One, Day Three		
Food	1,800 calories	2,000 calories
BREAKFAST		
Whole wheat toast	1 slice	1 slice
2% low-fat cottage cheese	1/2 cup	1/2 cup
Tub margarine	1 tablespoon	1 tablespoon
Sliced strawberries	1 cup	1 cup
Calcium-enriched orange juice	1 cup	1 cup
MORNING SNACK		
Fruited low-fat yogurt	1/2 cup	1/2 cup
LUNCH		
Ham sandwich: 3 ounces lean ham, 1 slice American cheese, 2 slices whole wheat bread, 2 romaine lettuce leaves, 2 teaspoons low-fat mayonnaise	1	Use 1 tablespoon mayonnaise
Skim milk	1 cup	1 cup
Green bell pepper, sliced, with 2 tablespoons fat-free ranch dressing for dip	1 serving	1 serving

Week One, Day Three (continued)		
Food	1,800 *calories*	2,000 *calories*
AFTERNOON SNACK		
Mint iced tea	As desired	As desired
Fresh orange	1 each	1 each
DINNER		
Italian Chicken and Rice	1 serving of recipe as shown	1 serving of recipe as shown
Spinach-carrot salad: 2 cups spinach, 1 shredded carrot, 2 tablespoons olive oil, 1 tablespoon balsamic vinegar	omit	1 serving
Apricots	3	3
EVENING SNACK		
Hot herbal tea	As desired	As desired
Nonfat vanilla frozen yogurt	1 cup	1 cup
Fresh raspberries	1 cup	1 cup
NUTRITION TOTALS FOR DAY THREE		
Calories	1,743	2,056
Fat (g)	32	61
Carbohydrate (g)	256	269
Protein (g)	115	116
Fiber (g)	34	37
Calories from fat (%)	16	26

Week One, Day Four		
Food	1,800 *calories*	2,000 *calories*
BREAKFAST		
Whole wheat toast	2 slices	2 slices
Peanut butter	2 tablespoons	2 tablespoons
Favorite jam	1 tablespoon	1 tablespoon
Skim milk	1 cup	1 cup

Food	1,800 calories	2,000 calories
MORNING SNACK		
Fresh orange	1	1
LUNCH		
Tuna Tomato Stack (page 124)	Recipe as shown	Recipe as shown
Apple	1	1
Skim milk	1 cup	1 cup
AFTERNOON SNACK		
Vegetable juice cocktail with fresh lime juice	1 cup	1 cup
Whole wheat bagel	1	1
Fat-free cream cheese	2 tablespoons	2 tablespoons
DINNER		
One Pot Chili	$^1/_{10}$ recipe	$^1/_{10}$ recipe
Steamed broccoli (1 cup) with 1 tablespoon fat-free ranch dressing and 2 teaspoons margarine	1 serving, omit margarine	1 serving
Chocolate chip cookies	2	2
Skim milk	$^1/_2$ cup	1 cup
EVENING SNACK		
Caffé latte	1 cup favorite coffee with 1 cup hot skim milk	1 cup favorite coffee with 1 cup hot skim milk
NUTRITION TOTALS FOR DAY FOUR		
Calories	1,833	1,977
Fat (g)	49	53
Carbohydrate (g)	255	277
Protein (g)	110	115
Fiber (g)	37	37
Calories from fat (%)	23	23

Week One, Day Five		
Food	1,800 calories	2,000 calories
BREAKFAST		
Oatmeal (½ cup oats cooked with 1 cup skim milk according to package directions)	1 serving	1 serving
Banana	1	1
Chopped walnuts	Omit	2 tablespoons for oatmeal
Orange juice	½ cup	½ cup
Coffee	As desired	As desired
MORNING SNACK		
Hot herbal tea	As desired	As desired
Fresh orange	1	1
LUNCH		
Tomato Turkey Stack (page 123)	Recipe as shown	Recipe as shown
American cheese	1 slice for sandwich	1 slice for sandwich
Skim milk	1 cup	1 cup
AFTERNOON SNACK		
Thin pretzel sticks	10	10
DINNER		
Chicken and Zucchini Spaghetti	¼ recipe	¼ recipe
Ice cream	½ cup	1 cup
EVENING SNACK		
Fresh peach, sliced, with 1 teaspoon brown sugar	1 serving	1 serving
Skim milk	1 cup	1 cup
NUTRITION TOTALS FOR DAY FIVE		
Calories	1,806	2,020
Fat (g)	36	51
Carbohydrate (g)	282	300
Protein (g)	95	99
Fiber (g)	26	26
Calories from fat (%)	18	22

Food	Week One, Day Six	
	1,800 calories	2,000 calories
BREAKFAST		
Creamy Breakfast Barley with Bananas and Dried Cranberries	Recipe as shown	Recipe as shown
Apple juice	omit	1 cup
MORNING SNACK		
Fresh orange	1	1
LUNCH		
Peanut butter and jelly sandwich: 2 slices whole wheat bread, 2 tablespoons peanut butter, and 1 tablespoon jam	1 serving	1 serving
Baby carrots (10) with 2 tablespoons fat-free French dressing as dip	1 serving	1 serving
Skim milk	¹/₂ cup	1 cup
AFTERNOON SNACK		
Fat-free fig bars	2	2
Skim milk	¹/₂ cup	¹/₂ cup
DINNER		
Hearty Vegetable Medley Soup	¹/₄ recipe	¹/₄ recipe
Salad made with 2 cups chopped romaine lettuce, ¹/₂ tomato, and 2 tablespoons regular favorite salad dressing	1 serving	1 serving
EVENING SNACK		
Fresh or frozen raspberries	1 cup	1 cup
Skim milk	¹/₂ cup	¹/₂ cup
NUTRITION TOTALS FOR DAY SIX		
Calories	1,803	1,963
Fat (g)	47	47
Carbohydrate (g)	300	335
Protein (g)	68	72
Fiber (g)	56	57
Calories from fat (%)	22	21

Week One, Day Seven		
Food	*1,800* *calories*	*2,000* *calories*
BREAKFAST		
High-fiber cereal (³/₄ cup) with ¹/₂ sliced banana and I tablespoon raisins	I serving	I serving
Skim milk	I cup	I cup
MORNING SNACK		
Blueberries	¹/₂ cup	I cup
LUNCH		
Pita Pocket Turkey Sandwich	Recipe as shown	Recipe as shown
Skim milk	1/2 cup	1/2 cup
Watermelon	I slice	2 slices
AFTERNOON SNACK		
Kiwi	I	I
Nonfat fruited yogurt	I cup	I cup
Seltzer water	As desired	As desired
DINNER		
Feta Cheese and Spinach Pizza	I serving	I serving
Skim milk	I cup	I cup
EVENING SNACK		
Strawberry shortcake: I slice angel food cake, ¹/₂ cup sliced strawberries, and I tablespoon nonfat whipped topping	I serving	I serving use 2 tablespoons nonfat whipped topping
NUTRITION TOTALS FOR DAY SEVEN		
Calories	1,771	1,956
Fat (g)	36	38
Carbohydrate (g)	272	316
Protein (g)	107	111
Fiber (g)	39	48
Calories from fat (%)	18	18

WEEK TWO: FOR THOSE WHO DO NOT CONTINUE TO TAKE XENICAL

Week Two, Day One

Food	1,800 calories	2,000 calories
BREAKFAST		
Whole-grain bagel	1	1
Low-fat cream cheese	2 tablespoons	2 tablespoons
Jam	1 tablespoon	1 tablespoon
Cantaloupe wedge	$1/4$ melon	$1/4$ melon
Skim milk	1 cup	1 cup
MORNING SNACK		
Calcium-fortified orange juice	1 cup	1 cup
LUNCH		
Vegetable Lentil Soup	$1/5$ recipe	$1/5$ recipe
Pita pocket salad: $1/2$ whole wheat pita pocket stuffed with $1/2$ cup romaine lettuce, $1/4$ cup chopped green onions, $1/4$ cup grated carrot, and drizzled with 1 tablespoon of favorite salad dressing	1 serving	1 serving
Skim milk	1 cup	1 cup
AFTERNOON SNACK		
Banana–mandarin orange salad made with 1 sliced banana and 1 cup drained canned mandarin oranges	1 serving	1 serving
Frozen nonfat whipped topping	1 tablespoon	$1/4$ cup
DINNER		
Grilled orange roughy topped with herb butter (garlic and chives sautéed in 1 teaspoon butter)	3 ounces fish	5 ounces fish
Cilantro–brown rice (stir 1 tablespoon freshly chopped cilantro into brown rice just before serving)	$1/2$ cup	1 cup
Steamed zucchini (1 cup) and tomatoes ($1/2$ cup)	1 serving	1 serving

Food	1,800 calories	2,000 calories
	EVENING SNACK	
Fresh fruit and cottage cheese salad: $1/2$ cup cantaloupe, $1/2$ cup watermelon, 1 kiwi, topped with $1/2$ cup nonfat extra-calcium cottage cheese	1 serving	1 serving
	NUTRITION TOTALS FOR DAY ONE	
Calories	1,787	1,972
Fat (g)	29	31
Carbohydrate (g)	303	330
Protein (g)	90	103
Fiber (g)	46	48
Calories from fat (%)	14	14

	Week Two, Day Two	
Food	1,800 calories	2,000 calories
	BREAKFAST	
Low-fat granola cereal	$1/2$ cup	1 cup
Fresh or frozen raspberries	$1/2$ cup	$3/4$ cup
Skim milk	1 cup	1 cup
	MORNING SNACK	
Banana spread with 1 tablespoon nonfat cream cheese blended with 1 teaspoon brown sugar and 1 tablespoon raisins	1 serving	1 serving
	LUNCH	
Vegetable-tuna pasta salad: $1/2$ cup cooked pasta shells, $1/2$ cup water-packed tuna, 5 quartered cherry tomatoes, 1 cup chopped broccoli, 1 chopped yellow sweet pepper, 2 tablespoons low-fat mayonnaise	1 serving	1 serving
Iced tea	As desired	As desired

Food	1,800 calories	2,000 calories

AFTERNOON SNACK

Food	1,800 calories	2,000 calories
¹/₂ cup fat-free chocolate sorbet sprinkled with 1 teaspoon chocolate sprinkles and 2 tablespoons fat-free frozen whipped topping	1 serving	1 serving

DINNER

Food	1,800 calories	2,000 calories
Portobello Burger	¹/₂ recipe	¹/₂ recipe
Steamed asparagus spears (5) with 1 teaspoon melted butter and lemon juice	1 serving	1 serving
1 fresh peach, sliced, with 1 cup skim milk	1 serving, use ¹/₂ cup skim milk	1 serving

EVENING SNACK

Food	1,800 calories	2,000 calories
3 cups air-popped popcorn sprinkled with 2 tablespoons fat-free Parmesan cheese	1 serving	1 serving
Orange juice spritzer: 1 cup iced lime seltzer water plus ¹/₄ cup iced orange juice	1 serving	1 serving

NUTRITION TOTALS FOR DAY TWO

	1,800 calories	2,000 calories
Calories	1,792	2,029
Fat (g)	47	51
Carbohydrate (g)	262	308
Protein (g)	94	102
Fiber (g)	30	34
Calories from fat (%)	23	22

Week Two, Day Three

Food	1,800 calories	2,000 calories

BREAKFAST

Food	1,800 calories	2,000 calories
Poached egg	1	2
Whole wheat bagel	¹/₂ small	¹/₂ small
Tub margarine	2 teaspoons	2 teaspoons
Skim milk	1 cup	1 cup
Fresh orange	1	1

Week Two, Day Three (continued)

Food	1,800 calories	2,000 calories
MORNING SNACK		
Fresh or frozen raspberries	¹/₂ cup	I cup
Nonfat coffee yogurt	¹/₂ cup	I cup
LUNCH		
Pita pocket ham sandwich: 3 ounces sliced ham and I slice American cheese stuffed into ¹/₂ whole wheat pita pocket with I tablespoon light mayonnaise	I serving	I serving
Apple, sliced, with ¹/₂ teaspoon cinnamon mixed with I teaspoon brown sugar	I serving	I serving
Skim milk	I cup	I cup
AFTERNOON SNACK		
Cantaloupe (¹/₄ melon sprinkled with fresh lime juice)	I serving	I serving
DINNER		
Rotini Chicken Salad with an Asian Peanut Sauce	¹/₂ recipe	¹/₂ recipe
Caffé latte: I cup hot skim milk mixed with I cup favorite flavored coffee	I serving	I serving
EVENING SNACK		
Favorite sliced veggies (2 cups) with dip of ¹/₄ cup nonfat sour cream mixed with ¹/₄ packet onion soup mix	I serving	I serving

NUTRITION TOTALS FOR DAY THREE

Calories	1,818	2,027
Fat (g)	48	55
Carbohydrate (g)	236	261
Protein (g)	120	133
Fiber (g)	32	36
Calories from fat (%)	23	24

Week Two, Day Four

Food	1,800 calories	2,000 calories
BREAKFAST		
Raisin bran cereal (1 cup) with sliced banana	1 serving	1 serving
Skim milk	1 cup	1 cup
MORNING SNACK		
Small whole-grain bagel with 1 tablespoon favorite jam	1 serving	1 serving
LUNCH		
Easy Garbanzo-Sunflower Salad	Recipe as shown	Recipe as shown
Low-fat fruited yogurt	1 cup	1 cup
Iced tea	As desired	As desired
AFTERNOON SNACK		
Vegetable juice cocktail	1 cup	1 cup
Oat bran pretzels	Omit	2 ounces
DINNER		
Beef tenderloin, broiled	3 ounces	3 ounces
Baked medium potato with 2 teaspoons margarine	1 serving	1 serving
Parslied Broccoli and Carrots	Recipe as shown	Recipe as shown
Whole wheat dinner roll with 1 teaspoon light margarine	1 serving	1 serving
EVENING SNACK		
Sliced strawberries (1 cup) with 1 cup skim milk and 1 teaspoon brown sugar	1 serving	1 serving

NUTRITION TOTALS FOR DAY FOUR

	1,800 calories	2,000 calories
Calories	1,798	2,025
Fat (g)	34	38
Carbohydrate (g)	307	351
Protein (g)	91	96
Fiber (g)	46	50
Calories from fat (%)	16	16

Week Two, Day Five		
Food	1,800 calories	2,000 calories
BREAKFAST		
Rye bagel	1 small	1 small
50% reduced-fat cheddar cheese (melted over bagel in a microwave or under a broiler)	2 ounces	2 ounces
MORNING SNACK		
Dried cranberries	Omit	2 tablespoons
Orange juice	1 cup	1 cup
LUNCH		
Italian Sub	Recipe as shown	Add 1 ounce low-fat American cheese
Skim milk	1 cup	1 cup
Peanut butter and chocolate banana: 1 banana, sliced lengthwise, spread with 1 tablespoon peanut butter and sprinkled with 1 tablespoon mini chocolate chips	1 serving	1 serving
AFTERNOON SNACK		
Fat-free fruited sorbet	1 cup	1 cup
DINNER		
Roasted chicken	3 ounces, without skin	3 ounces, without skin
Wild Rice with Mushrooms	$^1/_2$ recipe	$^1/_2$ recipe
Brussels sprouts (1 cup), sprinkled with freshly ground black pepper and balsamic vinegar	1 serving	1 serving
Skim milk	1 cup	1 cup
EVENING SNACK		
Baked Apple	Recipe as shown	Recipe as shown

NUTRITION TOTALS FOR DAY FIVE

Calories	1,828	1,983
Fat (g)	48	57
Carbohydrate (g)	255	268
Protein (g)	108	115
Fiber (g)	23	24
Calories from fat (%)	23	25

Week Two, Day Six

Food	1,800 calories	2,000 calories
BREAKFAST		
Hard-boiled egg	1	1
Whole wheat English muffin	1	1
Light tub margarine	1 tablespoon	1 tablespoon
Grapefruit juice	1 cup	1 cup
MORNING SNACK		
Blueberries	1 cup	1 cup
Nonfat vanilla yogurt	$1/2$ cup	1 cup
LUNCH		
Fast food: grilled chicken on bun, without mayonnaise and with double tomatoes and double lettuce	1 serving	1 serving
Fast-food side salad with 2 tablespoons of favorite regular dressing	1 serving	1 serving
Iced water	As desired	As desired
AFTERNOON SNACK		
Pretzel sticks	15	30
Peach nectar	1 cup	1 cup
DINNER		
Salsa-Seared Cod	Recipe as shown	Increase cod to 6 ounces
Basil-Tossed Rotini Pasta	$1/2$ recipe	$1/2$ recipe
Peas and carrots (use frozen for convenience)	1 cup	1 cup

Week Two, Day Six (continued)

Food	1,800 calories	2,000 calories
EVENING SNACK		
Mango sorbet (³/₄ cup) topped with ¹/₂ cup chopped papaya	I serving	I serving, use I cup sorbet
NUTRITION TOTALS FOR DAY SIX		
Calories	1,748	1,970
Fat (g)	52	52
Carbohydrate (g)	255	291
Protein (g)	80	97
Fiber (g)	23	23
Calories from fat (%)	26	23

Week Two, Day Seven

Food	1,800 calories	2,000 calories
BREAKFAST		
Broiled Mandarin Orange Breakfast Sandwich	Recipe as shown	Recipe as shown
Skim milk	Omit	¹/₂ cup
MORNING SNACK		
Low-fat fruited yogurt	¹/₂ cup	I cup
LUNCH		
Salmon Poppyseed Salad	Recipe as shown	Recipe as shown
Skim milk	Omit	¹/₂ cup
AFTERNOON SNACK		
Orange juice	I cup	I cup
DINNER		
Pork and Sweet Potatoes in a Rich Pear Sauce	¹/₂ recipe	¹/₂ recipe
Trail mix over sorbet: I tablespoon dry roasted sunflower seeds, I tablespoon chocolate chips, and 2 tablespoons packed raisins sprinkled over ¹/₂ cup fat-free chocolate sorbet	I serving	I serving

Food	1,800 calories	2,000 calories
	EVENING SNACK	
Fresh or frozen raspberries	¹/₂ cup	¹/₂ cup
Nonfat frozen yogurt	¹/₂ cup	¹/₂ cup
	NUTRITION TOTALS FOR DAY SEVEN	
Calories	1,826	2,017
Fat (g)	51	53
Carbohydrate (g)	243	271
Protein (g)	106	120
Fiber (g)	24	24
Calories from fat (%)	25	23

Recipes

FOR BREAKFAST

Broccoli, Mushroom, and Cheese Omelet

SERVES 1

1 egg
¹/₂ cup finely chopped raw broccoli
¹/₄ cup chopped mushrooms
1 ounce shredded sharp cheddar cheese

Heat a nonstick pan coated with vegetable oil spray over medium heat. Beat the egg slightly and pour into the hot pan. When the egg starts to congeal, add the vegetables and cheese. Cover and cook for 5 minutes, or until the egg is cooked and the cheese is melted. Remove the omelet from the pan and fold in half.

Per omelet: 196 calories, 14 grams fat, 4 grams carbohydrate, 14 grams protein, 1 gram fiber

Creamy Breakfast Barley with Bananas and Dried Cranberries

SERVES I

¼ cup medium uncooked pear barley
I cup skim milk
I teaspoon brown sugar
2 tablespoons dried cranberries
½ teaspoon vanilla extract
I banana, sliced

Combine the barley, milk, and brown sugar in a heavy saucepan. Simmer over low heat for 30 minutes. Add the cranberries and simmer 15 minutes more. Remove from the heat and stir in the vanilla and sliced banana.

Per serving: 429 calories, 2 grams fat, 90 grams carbohydrate, 15 grams protein, 11 grams fiber

Broiled Mandarin Orange Breakfast Sandwich

SERVES I

½ cup extra-calcium low-fat cottage cheese
I whole wheat English muffin
½ cup canned mandarin oranges, drained
I teaspoon sugar mixed with I teaspoon ground cinnamon

Spread the cottage cheese evenly on the muffin halves. Divide the orange segments between the halves. Sprinkle with the cinnamon-sugar mixture. Place on a broiler pan and broil for 2 or 3 minutes, or until the sugar bubbles.

Per serving: 279 calories, 3 grams fat, 48 grams carbohydrate, 21 grams protein, 7 grams fiber

FOR LUNCH

Tossed Shrimp Salad

SERVES 1

6 cold, cooked, peeled shrimp
$1/2$ cup chopped tomato
$1/4$ cup chopped green onions
$1/4$ cup grated carrots
1 tablespoon poppyseed dressing
1 cup chopped romaine lettuce

Toss all the ingredients except the romaine lettuce together. Place the salad on a bed of romaine lettuce and serve.

Per serving: 144 calories, 7 grams fat, 14 grams carbohydrate, 7 grams protein, 3 grams fiber

Favorite Tuna Pasta Salad

SERVES 4

2 cups cooked elbow macaroni
2 cans (6 ounces) chunk light tuna in water, drained
2 hard-boiled eggs, chopped
1 cup frozen petite peas, thawed
$1/4$ cup plus 2 tablespoons light Miracle Whip
$1/2$ cup chopped red onion
4 cups chopped romaine lettuce

Combine all the ingredients except the lettuce in a mixing bowl. Serve over the lettuce.

Per serving ($1/4$ of recipe): 356 calories, 10 grams fat, 33 grams carbohydrate, 33 grams protein, 4 grams fiber

Pita Pocket Turkey Sandwich

SERVES 1

1 whole wheat pita pocket
$1/2$ cup chopped romaine lettuce
$1/2$ cup chopped tomato
3 ounces lean turkey breast
$1/2$ ounce shredded Swiss cheese
1 tablespoon low-fat mayonnaise

Cut the top off the pita pocket. Stuff all the ingredients into the pita pocket.

Per serving: 411 calories, 12 grams fat, 42 grams carbohydrate, 37 grams protein, 6 grams fiber

Vegetable Lentil Soup

SERVES 5

2 tablespoons olive oil
1 cup chopped onion (about 2 small onions)
2 cloves garlic, chopped
1 can (28 ounces) crushed tomatoes
1 cup uncooked lentils
$1/4$ cup uncooked black beans
2 teaspoons beef bouillon granules or 2 cubes
3 cups water
$1/2$ teaspoon chili powder
$1/2$ teaspoon ground cumin
$1/4$ teaspoon ground black pepper
$1/4$ cup plus 2 tablespoons chopped fresh basil, divided
$1/4$ cup lemon juice, divided
8 ounces kale, chopped
8 ounces yellow zucchini, sliced
8 ounces green zucchini, sliced

Garnish:
2 medium tomatoes, chopped
5 tablespoons low-fat sour cream, divided

Heat the oil over medium heat. Add the onion and garlic, and sauté for 5 minutes to release the flavors.

Add the crushed tomatoes, lentils, black beans, bouillon, water, chili powder, cumin, and pepper. Cover the pan and simmer for 1 hour.

Uncover the pan and add the ¼ cup of basil, ⅛ cup lemon juice, kale, and yellow and green zucchini. Cover and simmer for 15 minutes.

Stir in the remaining basil and remaining lemon juice just before serving. Garnish with the chopped tomatoes and sour cream.

Per serving: 346 calories, 8 grams fat, 53 grams carbohydrate, 20 grams protein, 18 grams fiber

Easy Garbanzo-Sunflower Salad

SERVES 1

2 cups romaine lettuce
5 cherry tomatoes
½ cup garbanzo beans
2 tablespoons sunflower seeds
2 tablespoons reduced-fat Italian dressing

Combine all the ingredients in a small salad bowl.

Per serving: 282 calories, 10 grams fat, 40 grams carbohydrate, 12 grams protein, 10 grams fiber

Italian Sub

SERVES 1

2 ounces Italian bread, sliced lengthwise
2 ounces lean ham
1 ounce lean turkey salami
2 leaves romaine lettuce
3 thin tomato slices
1 tablespoon fat-free Italian dressing

Build the sandwich on 1 slice of Italian bread. Spread the dressing on the other slice of bread and place it on top.

Per serving: 305 calories, 8 grams fat, 33 grams carbohydrate, 24 grams protein, 3 grams fiber

Salmon Poppyseed Salad

SERVES 1

1 cup canned pink salmon (skin removed), flaked
1 tomato, chopped
½ cup chopped green onions
2 tablespoons regular poppyseed dressing
2 cups chopped fresh spinach

Combine all the ingredients except the spinach. Mix well with a fork. Arrange the spinach on a plate and place the salad mixture on top.

Per serving: 414 calories, 22 grams fat, 19 grams carbohydrate, 33 grams protein, 2 grams fiber

FOR DINNER

Buttered Rotini with Chicken Stir-Fry

SERVES 1

2 cloves garlic, minced
1-inch piece of fresh ginger, minced
1 teaspoon chicken bouillon granules
4 ounces boneless, skinless chicken breast, cut for stir-fry
1/2 cup chopped broccoli
1/4 cup chopped sweet red pepper
1/2 cup chopped sweet yellow pepper
1/4 cup sliced water chestnuts
1 1/2 cups cooked rotini pasta tossed with 2 teaspoons margarine

Coat a large nonstick pan with vegetable oil spray and heat over medium heat. Add the garlic, ginger, bouillon, and 1 tablespoon of water and cook for 4 minutes.

Raise the heat to high. Add the chicken and cook until it turns white on the outside.

Add the vegetables and water chestnuts, cover, and steam for 5 to 7 minutes, or until the chicken is thoroughly cooked and the vegetables are crisp-tender. Serve over pasta.

Per serving: 580 calories, 11 grams fat, 80 grams carbohydrate, 40 grams protein, 7 grams fiber

Italian Chicken and Rice

SERVES 4

1 pound boneless, skinless chicken breasts
1/2 cup chopped onion
1 can (28 ounces) crushed tomatoes with no salt added
3/4 cup dry (uncooked) brown rice
1 1/4 cups water
1 1/2 teaspoons oregano
1 teaspoon garlic salt
1 teaspoon parsley flakes
2 cups frozen cut okra
2 cups sliced mushrooms

Coat a large nonstick skillet with vegetable oil spray and heat to medium high. Add the chicken and onion, and sauté for 2 minutes per side, just to brown the chicken.

Add the tomatoes, rice, water, oregano, garlic salt, and parsley flakes. Stir well. Turn the heat to low, cover, and simmer for 20 minutes.

Uncover and add the okra and mushrooms. Cover and simmer 15 minutes more.

Per serving: 364 calories, 3 grams fat, 49 grams carbohydrate, 35 grams protein, 8 grams fiber

One Pot Chili

SERVES 10

1 pound ground sirloin
2 onions, chopped (about 2 cups)
2 stalks celery, chopped (about 1 cup)
2 cans (16 ounces) dark red kidney beans
1 can (28 ounces) no-salt-added crushed tomatoes
1 can (14½ ounces) no-salt-added whole tomatoes
2 teaspoons sugar
1 teaspoon dried sweet basil
1 teaspoon dried oregano
1 tablespoon chili powder
1 teaspoon salt
1 tablespoon garlic powder
¼ teaspoon ground black pepper

Coat the bottom of a heavy soup kettle with vegetable oil spray. Add the ground sirloin and onions, and brown on medium heat.

Stir in the remaining ingredients. Lower the heat and simmer, covered, for 45 minutes, allowing the flavors to reach their peak.

Per serving: 218 calories, 4 grams fat, 24 grams carbohydrate, 21 grams protein, 7 grams fiber

Chicken and Zucchini Spaghetti

SERVES 4

1 teaspoon light olive oil
2 medium onions, chopped
4 boneless, skinless chicken thighs, cut into chunks
8 ounces zucchini (about 1 medium)
8 ounces yellow summer squash (about 1 medium)
2 cups spicy red pepper pasta sauce
1/8 teaspoon salt
4 cups cooked thin spaghetti

Heat the oil over medium-high heat. Add the onions and chicken, and sauté until just slightly browned.

Lower the heat. Add the vegetables, salt, and pasta sauce. Simmer, covered, for 20 minutes, or until the vegetables are tender. Serve over the spaghetti.

Per serving: 390 calories, 8 grams fat, 54 grams carbohydrate, 24 grams protein, 7 grams fiber

Hearty Vegetable Medley Soup

SERVES 4

2 tablespoons light olive oil
3 cloves garlic, or to taste, sliced
1/2 red onion, chopped
4 cups water
4 carrots, peeled and sliced on the diagonal
2 medium potatoes, peeled and thinly sliced or diced
1 cup lentils, uncooked
1 teaspoon salt
1/4 teaspoon black pepper
1/2 teaspoon dried sweet basil
1 bag (1 pound) frozen mustard greens

Heat the oil over medium-low heat. Add the garlic and onion, and sauté for 10 minutes (to let the oil acquire the flavor of the garlic and onion).

Add the remaining ingredients except the mustard greens. Simmer, covered, for 50 minutes. The potatoes should cook and then break up (turn to mush) to thicken the soup.

Stir in the mustard greens and simmer 10 minutes more.

Per serving (1/4 of recipe): 350 calories, 8 grams fat, 56 grams carbohydrate, 19 grams protein, 22 grams fiber

Feta Cheese and Spinach Pizza

SERVES 3

Crust:

¹/₂ cup warm water

1 teaspoon dry yeast

1 teaspoon sugar

1 tablespoon olive oil

1 teaspoon salt

1 ¹/₃ cups all-purpose flour

Topping:

1 can (8 ounces) tomato sauce

2 teaspoons dried oregano

1 teaspoon garlic powder

2 teaspoons dried basil

1 medium onion, chopped

1 package (10 ounces) frozen spinach, thawed and drained

8 ounces mushrooms, sliced

1 jar (7.25 ounces) roasted red peppers, drained and cut into 1-inch pieces

3 ounces shredded part-skim mozzarella

5 ounces crumbled feta cheese

To make the crust: combine the water, yeast, and sugar, mixing well. Add the oil and salt, and mix well. Stir in the flour with a wooden spoon and beat until well blended, then beat an additional 20 strokes. (Alternatively, combine all the ingredients except the flour in a free-standing mixer and mix with the beater attachment until blended. Add 1 cup of flour and mix until blended. Switch to the dough hook, add the remaining flour, and beat for 2 minutes.)

Coat a 9-inch pizza pan with vegetable oil spray. Place the dough in the center of the pan and pat out until it covers the entire pan. Let rest for 10 minutes while you prepare the other ingredients.

Preheat the oven to 425 degrees. Spread the tomato sauce evenly over the dough. Sprinkle the spices evenly over the sauce. Add the vegetables in the order given. Sprinkle the mozzarella cheese evenly over the vegetables and top with the feta cheese.

Bake for 18 to 22 minutes, or until the cheese is slightly brown and the crust is crisp.

Per serving (¹/₃ of pizza): 563 calories, 19 grams fat, 70 grams carbohydrate, 29 grams protein, 9 grams fiber

Portobello Burger

SERVES 2

3 tablespoons balsamic vinegar

2 tablespoons olive oil

1 tablespoon freshly chopped basil

1 clove garlic, crushed

ground black pepper

2 teaspoons sugar

2 large portobello mushroom caps, washed and patted dry

6 ounces very lean ground sirloin

salt to taste

4 teaspoons nonfat blue cheese dressing

2 whole-grain hamburger buns

2 thick tomato slices

2 large leaves romaine lettuce

In a shallow container, mix the vinegar, oil, basil, garlic, ¼ teaspoon pepper, and sugar. Add the mushroom caps, top side down. Spoon the liquid on the bottom of the caps. Cover and marinate for 1 hour at room temperature or overnight in the refrigerator.

Add salt and pepper to the ground sirloin and shape into 2 patties. Grill for 5 minutes on one side, then turn over. Add the mushroom caps to the grill or broiler pan, top side up (discard the marinade). Grill 5 minutes more, or until the mushrooms are slightly brown and the patties are no longer pink in the middle.

Build the portobello burger: place 1 teaspoon dressing on the bottom of the bun; add the patty, tomato slice, and mushroom cap. Place 1 teaspoon blue cheese dressing on top of the mushroom, and top with the bun.

Per serving: 480 calories, 23 grams fat, 37 grams carbohydrate, 33 grams protein, 5 grams fiber

Rotini Chicken Salad with an Asian Peanut Sauce

SERVES 2

6 ounces cooked chicken breast, cooled and cut into bite-sized pieces
$1/2$ cup chopped green onion tops
$11/2$ cups cooked rotini at room temperature
2 cups chopped romaine lettuce

Sauce:
3 tablespoons smooth peanut butter
3 tablespoons light soy sauce
2 teaspoons granulated sugar
$1/2$ cup fresh coriander (cilantro) leaves

Garnish:
1 large carrot, grated

In a small mixing bowl, combine the chicken, onion tops, and pasta.

Divide the chopped lettuce between 2 dinner plates. Divide the chicken-pasta mixture and place on top of the lettuce.

In a small food processor or blender, process the sauce ingredients until the cilantro is in tiny pieces. Drizzle half of the mixture over each serving. Sprinkle the grated carrot over each serving.

Per serving: 479 calories, 16 grams fat, 45 grams carbohydrate, 39 grams protein, 5 grams fiber

Parslied Broccoli and Carrots

SERVES 1

1 cup frozen broccoli pieces
1 cup frozen carrot coins
$1/4$ cup chopped fresh parsley
2 teaspoons balsamic vinegar

Combine the broccoli and carrots in a microwaveable container and cook according to package directions, until the vegetables are heated through. Add the parsley and vinegar, toss, and serve.

Per serving: 105 calories, 1 gram fat, 22 grams carbohydrate, 6 grams protein, 9 grams fiber

Wild Rice with Mushrooms

SERVES 2

2 cloves garlic, minced
4 teaspoons olive oil
2 cups sliced mushrooms
2 cups cooked wild rice
$1/2$ teaspoon salt
freshly ground black pepper to taste

Heat the garlic in the oil over low heat for 5 minutes, until the oil acquires the flavor of the garlic. Add the mushrooms and sauté for 3 to 5 minutes, until they wilt.

Stir in the rice and salt. Add the pepper and serve.

Per serving: 267 calories, 10 grams fat, 39 grams carbohydrate, 8 grams protein, 4 grams fiber

Salsa-Seared Cod

SERVES 1

Marinade:
1 tablespoon extra-virgin olive oil
2 cloves garlic, minced
1 tablespoon salsa

4 ounces cod fillet

Combine the marinade ingredients. Place the fish in the marinade and marinate for at least 2 hours in the refrigerator (overnight is okay).

Transfer the fish and marinade to a nonstick pan coated with vegetable oil spray. Simmer over medium heat for 15 minutes.

Remove the fish and cover to keep warm. Simmer the sauce for 5 minutes to thicken, or until reduced by about half. Serve the sauce over the fish.

Per serving: 226 calories, 14 grams fat, 3 grams carbohydrate, 21 grams protein, 0 fiber

Basil-Tossed Rotini Pasta

SERVES 2

2 cups cooked rotini pasta
1 teaspoon extra-virgin olive oil mixed with 2 teaspoons balsamic vinegar
½ cup chopped fresh basil

Drizzle the oil-vinegar mixture over the pasta. Sprinkle on the chopped basil, toss, and serve immediately.

Per serving: 224 calories, 3.3 grams fat, 41 grams carbohydrate, 7 grams protein, 2.2 grams fiber

Pork and Sweet Potatoes in a Rich Pear Sauce

SERVES 2

1 teaspoon canola oil
½ cup chopped red onion
8 ounces very lean pork, cut for stir-fry
1 teaspoon salt
2 medium-sized sweet potatoes (about 12 to 14 ounces with peel), peeled and cut into ½-inch slices
1 cup pear nectar
¼ teaspoon black pepper
1 teaspoon dried thyme
1 large red pear, quartered, seeded, and each quarter halved

Sauté the onion in the oil over medium-high heat. Add the pork chunks and salt. Stir-fry for 2 or 3 minutes, or until the meat is slightly browned.

Add the sweet potatoes, pear nectar, pepper, and thyme, and mix well. Cover and let simmer for 30 minutes; the mixture should bubble gently.

Uncover, gently fold in the pear chunks, and simmer, uncovered, for 15 minutes, or until the liquid has reduced to about half and has thickened.

Per serving (½ of recipe): 573 calories, 12 grams fat, 67 grams carbohydrate, 40 grams protein, 8 grams fiber

FOR DESSERTS AND SNACKS

Baked Apple

SERVES 1

1 baking apple, cored
½ cup diet black cherry soda
1 cinnamon stick

Place the apple in a small baking dish. Pour the soda into the core and place the cinnamon stick in the core. Bake at 350 degrees for 30 minutes, or until the apple is soft.

Per serving: 81 calories, 0 grams fat, 21 grams carbohydrate, 0 grams protein, 4 grams fiber

Totally Decadent Banana Chocolate Chip Muffins

MAKES 18 MUFFINS

3 very ripe bananas
3 tablespoons olive oil
¼ cup applesauce
¾ cup granulated sugar
¼ cup nonfat plain yogurt
2 eggs
⅓ cup wheat germ
½ cup whole wheat flour
1¼ cups white flour
½ teaspoon baking soda
3 ounces mini chocolate chips

Preheat the oven to 350 degrees. Place the bananas, oil, applesauce, and sugar in a mixing bowl. Mix on medium speed until the bananas are pureed and the ingredients are well mixed. Add the yogurt, eggs, and wheat germ, and mix until blended.

In a small bowl, combine the flours, baking powder, and baking soda. Add to the wet ingredients and mix just until all the ingredients are well blended. Stir in the chocolate chips.

Coat 18 muffin cups with vegetable oil spray or line with paper liners. Divide the batter among the 18 cups. Bake for 22 to 28 minutes, or until a knife inserted in the center comes out clean.

Per muffin: 155 calories, 5 grams fat, 25 grams carbohydrate, 3 grams protein, 2 grams fiber

The Maintenance Program on Your Own

We have created two weeks of fabulous menus and recipes for you to make your maintenance program interesting, easy and enjoyable. Perhaps, though, you would like to create your own menus, as you may have done during the weight loss portion of this program. As you learned in chapter 5, use the table below and choose the number of servings from each food category that corresponds to the calorie level you are following for maintenance. Refer to the *What Is in a Serving?* information on pages 142–143 for serving sizes. And remember that the only way the maintenance program works is if you adhere carefully to the serving sizes listed.

Food	1,800 calories	2,000 calories
BREAKFAST (NUMBER OF SERVINGS)		
Protein food	1	1
Grain food	2	2
Fruit	1	1
Dairy	1	1
Added fat	2	2
LUNCH (NUMBER OF SERVINGS)		
Protein food	2	3
Grain food	2	3
Vegetable	2	2
Fruit	1	1
Dairy	1	1
Added fat	2	2
DINNER (NUMBER OF SERVINGS)		
Protein food	3	4
Grain food	3	3
Vegetable	3	3
Fruit	1	2
Added fat	2	2
SNACK FOODS (NUMBER OF SERVINGS)		
Grain food	1	2
Vegetable	2	2
Fruit	3	3
Dairy	2	2

Keeping Records—Your Personal Food Diary

Because we know that keeping weight off can be just as difficult as losing it in the first place, it is important to continue to keep track of what you eat. If you are still taking Xenical, this becomes even more necessary, since we urge that you still consume no more that 20 fat grams at any meal. Whether you are creating your own menus or following ours, use this food diary to record what you eat, to calculate total calories, and to track fat grams for each meal. Our photocopiable chart is also a useful tool for planning your daily menus. Refer to "Monitoring Fat: Guidelines and Tables" on pages 144–150 of chapter 5 for more information on the fat and calorie content of food servings.

My Food Diary

Meal	Food Eaten	Serving Size	Number of Calories	Number of Fat Grams	Total Number of Fat Grams for the Meal (Not to Exceed 20 Grams)
Breakfast					
Lunch					
Dinner					
Snacks					
Total Daily Fat and Calories					

How to Avoid Gaining Back Lost Weight

You're human. Acknowledging this essential fact is the first step to not regaining the weight you've lost with the Xenical diet and exercise plan.

This acknowledgment cuts two important ways. Most important, you need to recognize that you lost the weight with your human efforts, not because a pill gave you superhuman powers. At the same time, you are not perfect, which means you will have moments when you do what every other human being does: you will eat foods you enjoy, in amounts greater than you should.

Changing dietary habits is one of the most difficult tasks you will ever accomplish. You still have to eat and therefore are constantly exposed to temptation.

I'd like to share with you the secrets I've both learned from my patients and have taught to others. None is more important than another, and they all work well together to help you maintain your new, healthier weight.

Have a Plan. Decide ahead of time how you will cope with slip-ups. This is an extension of the "I'm human" acknowledgment. It cannot be emphasized strongly enough that how you react to slipping up determines where you go after the slip-up. Although it is very common to feel defeated and guilty and to tell yourself you've been "bad," these negative feelings and the resultant self-chastisement can be very damaging. They often lead to further overeating. Focusing on the guilt may turn one measly candy bar from the grocery store checkout line into an ice cream–pizza–fast-food binge.

You have two choices as you think about how you will deal with a slip-up:

1. You can learn from your mistake. This is *the ideal solution.* I call it falling forward or prolapsing. For example, learn to grocery-shop right after you've eaten a meal, when candy bars aren't so tempting. You can also select the candy-free checkout line (most grocery stores have them now).

2. You can feel guilty and continue overeating, which I call falling backward. We also call this a relapse. You might feel so guilty, for example, that when you stop for gas after getting groceries, you buy three more candy bars and eat them. Obviously, this isn't a

good response. This sometimes leads to total collapse, where the overeating goes on for days.

Included in the advice I give my clients to help them deal with small prolapses—and prevent those from becoming relapses or collapses—is that they tally the calories in the one item eaten that wasn't on the plan. A cookie might be 100 calories and a candy bar 200; as part of the big picture, those few calories aren't worth relapsing or collapsing.

Understand the Difference Between Hunger and Appetite. Hunger is the real physical need for food; it is often accompanied by a gnawing feeling in the pit of the stomach and audible rumbling. Appetite, on the other hand, is the desire to eat something, and it often has little to do with whether or not you're hungry. Without a healthy appetite, of course, you would have a hard time eating enough to stay alive. But too often appetite activates in response to external cues, causing us to eat when we're not hungry. These are some of the external cues you have to learn to control to prevent regaining weight:

- The clock: do you eat just because the clock says 12 noon or 6 P.M.? Instead, tune in to what your stomach says.
- Social situations: do you always have popcorn at the movies or indulge in the dessert cart at your favorite restaurant? Find a way to deal with these external cues, especially if there are several of them. Remember, when you say that "it's just when I go out," to ask yourself how many special situations you give in to in a month's time.
- The vending machines at work: these glass-encased goody boxes are notorious external cues, especially in the afternoon when energy is low and frustration is high. If you must, empty the change and dollar bills out of your wallet and leave the money in the car.

Ask Yourself if You Use Food as a Tranquilizer. You are not alone if you have used food to bring out good feelings or block bad ones. Learning to control this, though, is essential to keeping your weight off. If you were to analyze your eating behaviors, which I encourage you to do using the food diary earlier in this chapter, you would probably find that you eat certain foods in response to a specific negative feeling. But don't give food magical powers—which is what you might have been doing all those years before you lost weight. Food is calories and nutrients, not good feelings.

Plan for Risky Situations. One of my patients, Sally, repeatedly told me that she could stick to a lower-calorie eating plan if she didn't have a family birthday party or gathering. Over a couple of months I discovered that Sally had one of those huge (and, fortunately, happy) families where there were parties and gatherings nearly every weekend—and sometimes twice on one weekend. For Sally these represented risky eating situations. Everyone brought their favorite (and usually high-calorie) treats, which Sally had a hard time resisting. Although she dieted fairly successfully all week, the weekend's risky eating situations kept Sally from losing weight; in fact, she just kept gaining.

Over time, I helped Sally learn to live with these situations by planning for them. This meant deciding ahead of time what she was going to eat at these affairs. If she knew, for example, that Auntie Ann was going to bring her famous chocolate mayonnaise cake, she would plan to have a sliver of that and sip on club soda the rest of the evening. Because these family gatherings were constant, Sally had to deal with these foods by slivers and spoonfuls rather than by full portions.

Analyze how often you are put into risky eating situations and then plan accordingly.

Continue to Set Goals—Even After Reaching Your Goal Weight. Your goal weight is just one of the goals you have for your health—both mental and physical. Continue to set goals for healthy eating, exercising (not to sound like a broken record), cooking nutritious food, and being proud of yourself for resisting temptation. Don't set impossible goals, but do set ambitious ones that are just a little beyond your reach. Balance is key here. If your goals are too difficult, you may give up early in the game. But if they're too easy, you may not stick with the program because you'll be so confident that you can achieve them without working.

Overall, setting small goals helps you know where you are going and whether you are on the right track. Otherwise, you struggle with trying to make a lot of changes at one time and end up feeling overwhelmed. Setting goals makes weight loss and weight maintenance easier for another reason: it's a great source of self-motivation. When you decide on definite goals, you make a commitment to yourself that you'll work hard to accomplish your final objective of weighing less and being healthier. The more defined the goals, the more likely you are to achieve them.

Understand Stress Eating. I treat this type of eating separately because it is such a common cause of overeating. Unfortunately, food does work in the short term to make you feel better when you are under stress. Ultimately, it causes even more stress. Learn to associate calming stress with something other than food. For example, take a hot bath, go for a walk, or enjoy a spin on the exercise bike. Even just a few moments of slow, deep breathing is a great destressor. Make the mental association with these nonfood destressors and conjure it up again and again. It will work for you—I know it can.

Put Away Temptation. I call this the clean kitchen approach. Does the cookie jar or the bread basket call your name? What about the bowl of candy you have out for the grandchildren? Put all these things away (or just get rid of them altogether). Instead, decorate your table and countertops with fresh flowers every week from the grocery store. Yes, you're worth it.

Freeze an Overeating Moment. Stop mid-bite and ask yourself what you are doing and if you really want to do it. Then pat yourself on the back as you walk away. You've now turned a negative moment into a positive one. There is no need to chastise yourself for taking that bite, because you stopped yourself. Take these wonderfully successful moments and run with them. You'll only be more successful next time.

Forgive Yourself and Recover. Whether it was the excellent company, the two glasses of wine, or just being caught up in the party atmosphere, you ended up eating to the point that your clothes felt a size smaller than when you put them on. All is not lost, though, if you allow yourself to recover rather than punish yourself with more overeating. When you arrive home, look at yourself in the mirror and say, "I forgive you. It's time to put the mistake to rest and move on to healthier thoughts." Awake the next day and start over as if the digression never occurred, rather than punishing yourself by continuing to eat out of control or starving yourself to the point of bingeing again.

Don't Undereat. Whether you are trying to lose weight or keep off lost weight, undereating can make you overeat. Constant restraint and self-denial generally leads people to binge on something they've made themselves "stay away from." To avoid this starve-crave-binge cycle, eat regular meals and snacks. As old-fashioned at it sounds, a good breakfast is at the top of the eating priority list.

Give Up Your Membership in the Clean Plate Club. Like most people, you probably start at least some meals with true physical hunger. But then, also like most people, you sometimes forget to check in with your hunger barometer, eating instead according to external signals and swabbing your plate clean. Do you have a second portion at dinner just because it's sitting in front of you on the table? These powerful social and visual cues can keep you eating long past the time you were truly satisfied—and will foil weight-loss and weight-maintenance attempts. The best advice: try always to leave at least one bite of everything on your plate, just to help you remember to eat only what you are hungry for.

Get the Help You Need. For some people, close contact with a weight-loss counselor is key to weight-loss success. The individualized support and creative problem solving that counselors offer are just what some people need. You are worth the expense if that is what you need. Just be sure to find a reputable weight-loss expert, using your physician as a resource when necessary.

Check Up on Yourself. The weight-loss diary you used to help you lose weight will be your best friend for life. Research clearly reveals that people who track what they eat are more successful at weight loss. You don't need to track daily eating after you lose weight, but I do recommend writing down what you eat once or twice a week. If you start to regain, go back to daily tracking. You'll be amazed at how quickly the pounds will come off again.

Plan Ahead. Don't leave eating to chance even after you've lost weight. Plan a week or two of menus at a time, which also makes shopping and cooking easier; you can make big batches of favorite recipes and repeat them.

Weigh Yourself Weekly. I don't want you to focus on the scale, but you do need to know how you are doing. Tracking your weight is one way to do so. Weigh yourself once a week on the same day and at the same time, and keep a diary of these weights. If you start to see a trend toward gaining, then slip back into your weight-loss mode: return to the calorie level on which you lost weight. Be wary of those times when you steer clear of the scale. I know from experience that people who do that know they are gaining and don't want to acknowledge it.

Stay Well Hydrated. It's no secret that people who drink more water have an easier time keeping weight off. The reasons are multiple and complex, but the most important thing is that drinking water works.

One very important fact: we often mistake thirst for hunger, which causes us to go rummaging through cupboards when a trip to the kitchen faucet would have solved the problem. If you don't like water "straight up," then do whatever it takes to drink more. Put limes or lemons in water, drink bottled water, or simply refrigerate sipper bottles of water. An easy way to make sure you get all the water you need is to buy four 20-ounce sipper bottles and fill them every night for the next day.

While it's no secret that weight loss is very difficult, many people do not realize that keeping weight off is just as challenging. Use the meal plans and the other advice I have given you in this chapter to help you meet the challenge and stay slimmer for life.

8

Safety Concerns

Your safety comes first. No matter how much you want to or need to lose weight, you may be one of the people who should not take Xenical. In any event, you should consult your physican to determine whether Xenical is safe for you. It may not be if you take certain medications, which may interact with Xenical in your body. If you do take Xenical, you must follow all the guidelines so that you avoid the problems that can result from taking it incorrectly. This chapter helps you understand these points. We'll also discuss two matters that have been studied thoroughly: how Xenical affects vitamin absorption and its relationship to breast cancer.

When You Should Not Take Xenical

When you visit your physician to get the prescription for Xenical, discuss all your current medical conditions as well as your past medical history, especially if the prescribing doctor is someone other than your regular family physician. To repeat what was said in chapter 2: it is important that you do not take Xenical if:

- you have a chronic malabsorption condition, meaning that your gastrointestinal tract does not absorb nutrients as well as it should—for example, if you have Crohn's disease or have had some of your bowel surgically removed;
- you have cholestasis, or blocked bile ducts;

- you have had an allergic reaction to Xenical;
- you are pregnant or nursing;
- you are younger than eighteen or older than sixty-five; Xenical has not yet been tested in these younger and older age groups, so recommendations cannot be made for these people.

When to Use Xenical Cautiously (or Maybe Not at All)

If you have any chronic medical condition or take certain medications, be sure to discuss these matters with the physician who prescribes Xenical for you. There may be certain instances when drug interactions could occur, or perhaps the drug could affect your medical condition adversely.

A drug interaction means that certain drugs don't mix well in the body. Only your physician can determine whether you might experience a potentially unsafe drug interaction when you take Xenical in combination with other medications. This might occur with prescription drugs but can also happen with over-the-counter medications and even herbal remedies.

Some of the things doctors know about Xenical and how it affects other drugs are included below. This list is by no means complete; it is imperative that you discuss all medications you take with the physician who prescribes Xenical for you.

The makers of Xenical recommend caution if you are taking cyclosporine, a strong medication used to change how the immune system works. This drug is also known as Sandimmune, Ciclosporin, and Cyclosporin A. Since changes in cyclosporine absorption into the body have been reported with changes in people's diets, caution is needed when deciding whether or not to take Xenical.

Caution is also advised if you take pravastatin, also called Pravachol, a medication used to lower blood cholesterol levels. A study was done of twenty-four patients who took pravastatin and Xenical, all of whom had high cholesterol levels. The researchers found that Xenical was additive to the cholesterol-lowering effect of pravastatin—that is, Xenical caused the pravastatin to work better than it would without Xenical—resulting in higher blood levels of pravastatin than would normally be expected. Blood levels of pravastatin in those taking both drugs were increased about 30 percent over those taking pravastatin but not taking Xenical.

Another drug that might not mix well with Xenical is warfarin, a blood thinning drug that is also known as Coumadin. Regulating the amount of vitamin K in the bloodstream is important when taking this medication because vitamin K affects blood thinning, too. Studies show that when people take Xenical, vitamin K absorption may be decreased (because it is a fat-soluble vitamin), and therefore blood levels of vitamin K tend to drop. The makers of Xenical recommend that people who take warfarin and who are prescribed Xenical should be monitored closely for changes in coagulation parameters, or blood tests that show how thin the blood is.

This list of drug interactions and cautions is by no means complete. Be sure to discuss any and all medications you take with the physician who prescribes Xenical, including over-the-counter or nonprescription medications as well as herbal and other natural remedies.

The makers of Xenical also recommend cautious use by those who have a history of high levels of urinary oxalate (a chemical substance in the urine) and/or certain kinds of kidney stones. This is because some people who take Xenical may develop high levels of urinary oxalate and may be at risk for developing kidney stones.

One other note of caution, although a positive one indeed: as noted in chapter 2, using Xenical and losing weight can improve the blood glucose, or blood sugar, tests of people with diabetes. It is important to monitor blood sugars very carefully while using Xenical. In some cases, blood sugars may improve to such an extent that it may be necessary to lower the dose of insulin or other medications used to control diabetes. Consult your diabetes care specialist on this important task, and on the dietary and exercise changes you are making, so that you can avoid episodes of hypoglycemia (your blood sugar level dropping too low).

Taking Xenical Correctly

Because we're so concerned for your safety, we're going to be redundant here; we're going to repeat the information on taking Xencial safely even though we've already covered it in previous chapters.

1. Take only the prescribed dose of Xenical. Your physician will prescribe 120-milligram Xenical tablets. The most effective dose is one 120-milligram tablet three times daily with meals.

2. Take Xenical at the correct time, which is at the beginning of the meal. With some medications it doesn't matter whether you take them on an empty or a full stomach. Not so with Xenical. The drug is designed to stop some of the fat in your meals from being absorbed, and in order to do this, it has to be in the intestinal tract

when you eat meals containing fat. It goes to work quickly to inhibit fat absorption.

3. If you are planning to dine out, don't take the pill before leaving the house because too much time may pass before you eat, and Xenical may lose its effectiveness before then. Like any pill, Xenical has a limited "therapeutic window," which is just a fancy way of saying that it works for only a limited time once inside the body.

4. Follow the diet properly, limiting yourself to the prescribed 30 percent of calories as fat. It is also strongly recommended that you not eat more than 20 fat grams at any one time. Some people have thought that because Xenical inhibits fat absorption, they can finally eat all the fat they want and suffer no consequences. But the consequences of eating too much fat while taking Xenical can be quite noticeable. You may experience intestinal gas, fecal urgency, and other gastrointestinal symptoms. It must be emphasized that if you take Xenical correctly and limit fat intake as we have indicated, you minimize the chance of experiencing these side effects.

About Fat-Soluble Vitamins

Because Xenical decreases fat absorption, it may also decrease the absorption of fat-soluble vitamins. Studies have shown that the levels of vitamin D and beta-carotene (a form of vitamin A that is found in fruits and vegetables) may be low in patients who take Xenical. During the early studies of Xenical, we measured the levels of these vitamins as well as other fat-soluble ones in the bloodstream of patients taking Xenical. These patients were not on vitamin supplements. For comparison, we also measured the vitamin levels in patients who took the placebo; this gave us an opportunity to understand how Xenical affected vitamin levels. According to these studies:

- 2.2 percent of patients who took Xenical had low blood levels of vitamin A, compared to 1.0 percent of those taking a placebo.
- 12.0 percent of patients who took Xenical had low blood levels of vitamin D, compared to 6.6 percent of those taking a placebo.
- 5.8 percent of patients who took Xenical had low blood levels of vitamin E, compared to 1.0 percent of those on a placebo.
- 6.1 percent of patients who took Xenical had low blood levels of beta-carotene, compared to 1.7 percent of those who took a placebo.

With these study results, we know that it is important for people taking Xenical to take a vitamin/mineral supplement that supplies 100 percent of the U.S. RDA for all essential nutrients. Don't take more vitamins, because you will simply excrete the excess. Also, take your vitamin/mineral supplement with one of your snacks or perhaps at bedtime for maximum absorption. Just be sure to take the supplement more than two hours before or after taking Xenical so that Xenical doesn't interfere with absorption of the vitamins. It doesn't matter what time of day you choose; just be consistent so that you don't forget.

About Breast Cancer and Xenical

As noted in chapter 1, Roche withdrew its New Drug Application for FDA approval of Xenical to study a particular finding, an imbalance in the number of breast cancers observed between the treatment and placebo groups in the clinical trials. Roche then studied all women who had ever received Xenical; the larger numbers gave them a better ability to detect problems. Roche ultimately found that these findings were simply due to chance, but it is worth going through the whole process to reassure you.

Fifteen cases of breast cancer were reported among the 1,642 women in the Xenical studies. Although early analysis suggested that Xenical probably was not responsible, the makers of Xenical took the most cautious approach and withdrew the New Drug Application until they could study the situation completely and thoroughly. Here's what they found.

Overall, it was determined that the total number of cases that may have emerged during the clinical trials and follow-up period was four: two in the treatment group and two in the placebo group. The remaining eleven of the fifteen cases diagnosed during the course of the clinical trials were classified as preexisting.

Out of 1,063 women over the age of forty-five years, ten of the twelve cases of breast cancer in the treatment group, or the women who took Xenical, were classified as existing prior to the initiation of the trial. The remaining two cases were classified as possibly emerging after the initiation of treatment.

Out of 579 women over the age of forty-five, one case of breast cancer in the placebo group, or the women who took the sugar pill, was classified as preexisting, and two were classified as possibly emerging after the initiation of treatment.

The researchers determined that in each group of women—those taking Xenical and those taking a placebo—there were possibly two cases of breast cancer that emerged after starting treatment. Overall, there was no evidence that Xenical, or any products that it forms in the body after it is metabolized, causes or stimulates the growth of breast cancer. Some other evidence that leads Xenical scientists to the conclusion that the drug does not cause breast cancer include:

- Animal studies do not indicate any carcinogenic potential with Xenical. Xenical's low (less than 1 percent) absorption into the body from the gastrointestinal tract and its lack of estrogen-stimulating effects lend additional support to the conclusion that no known biological association exists between Xenical and breast cancer.
- In animal studies there was no stimulation of normal breast tissue, nor was there evidence for enhanced growth or earlier onset of spontaneously occurring breast tumors in rodents.
- The histologic appearance, or how the tumor cells looked under the microscope, of the breast tumors found in the Xenical studies varied. In other words, there wasn't just one type of breast cancer tumor cell, which one would expect if the Xenical were responsible for the breast cancer.
- By looking under the microscope at breast cancer cells, scientists can also tell how long the cells have been growing. Examining the breast cancer cases under the microscope provided unequivocal evidence that the vast majority of breast cancer cases existed prior to the women's enrolling in the study.

Because it is so important, we restate what we said in chapter 1: a comprehensive review of the study data found that the additional cases of breast cancer had nothing to do with the Xenical and were simply a matter of chance. In November 1997, Roche resubmitted its New Drug Application with analyses of the breast cancer data. Based on this scientific evidence, Roche doesn't believe that Xenical is an initiator or stimulator of breast cancer or tumors associated with breast cancer. Xenical's NDA again received accelerated review status from the FDA and was ultimately approved.

Overall Safety

For your own personal well-being, don't ignore even one of the safety factors discussed in this chapter. Your good health depends on it. If you cannot take Xenical for some reason, then try the diet and exercise plan in this book. Although they are tailored for use with Xenical, our programs are suitable for all who want to lose weight and improve their health.

During the twenty-five years I have been helping men and women lose weight, I have seen so many people looking for assistance in their struggle to be healthier. Xenical offers such assistance, increasing the rate at which people can lose pounds and at the same time helping them adopt a low-fat eating plan they can adhere to in the long term. If you have chosen to take Xenical, I wholeheartedly encourage you to follow carefully the instructions in this book to lose weight safely and keep it off. I wish you better health for life, with the Xenical advantage.

References

American Cancer Society. *1996 Dietary Guidelines.* September 1996.

American Heart Association. 1997 *Heart and Stroke Statistical Update.* Dallas, TX.

Anderson, J. W., et al. 1995. "Meta-Analysis of the Effects of Soy Protein Intake on Serum Lipids." *New England Journal of Medicine.* 333: 276–82.

Appel, L. H. 1997. "A Clinical Trial of the Effects of Dietary Patterns on Blood Pressure." *New England Journal of Medicine.* 336: 1117–24.

"Are Reduced-Fat Foods Keeping Americans Healthier?" *Tufts University Health & Nutrition Letter.* 1998. 16 (1): 4–5.

Arnow, B., J. Kenardy and W. S. Agras. 1995. "The Emotional Eating Scale: The Development of a Measure to Assess Coping with Negative Affect by Eating." *International Journal of Eating Disorders.* 18: 79–90.

Aronne, L. J., et al. *Weigh Less, Live Longer: Dr. Lou Aronne's "Getting Healthy" Plan for Permanent Weight Control.* New York: John Wiley and Sons, 1995.

Aylett, M. 1996. "Use of Home Blood Pressure Measurements to Diagnose 'White Coat Hypertension' in General Practice." *Journal of Human Hypertension.* 10: 17–20.

Ballor, Douglas, et al. 1990. "Exercise Intensity Does Not Affect the Composition of Diet and Exercise Induced Body Mass Loss." *American Journal of Clinical Nutrition.* 51: 142–46.

Barch, D. H., et al. 1996. "Structure-Function Relationships of the Dietary Anticarcinogen Ellagic Acid." *Carcinogenesis.* 17: 265–69.

Berdanier, C. D. *Advanced Nutrition: Micronutrients.* New York: CRC Press, 1998.

Berg, F. M. 1996. "Dysfunctional Eating: A New Concept." *Healthy Weight Journal.* September/October: 88–94.

Blank, D. M., and R. D. Mattes. 1990. "Sugar and Spice: Similarities and Sensory Attributes." *Nursing Research.* 39 (5): 290–93.

Bostick, R. M., et al. 1993. "Reduced Risk of Colon Cancer with High Intake of Vitamin E: The Iowa Women's Health Study." *Cancer Research.* 53: 4230–37.

Bots, M. L., et al. 1997. "Common Carotid Intima-Media Thickness and Risk of Stroke and Myocardial Infarction: The Rotterdam Study." *Circulation.* 96: 1432–37.

Brownell, K. D. *The LEARN Program for Weight Control.* Philadelphia: University of Pennsylvania Press, 1989.

Carmody, T. P., et al. 1995. "Dietary Helplessness and Distribution in Weight Cyclers and Maintainers." *International Journal of Eating Disorders.* 18 (3): 247–56.

Cirilla, D. 1993. "Cravings Studies Provide Valuable but Incomplete Information." *Chittar's Food Engineering.* 65 (12): 26.

Davidson, M. H., et al. 1999. "Weight Control and Risk Factor Reduction in Obese Subjects Treated for Two Years with Orlistat." *Journal of the American Medical Association.* 281: 235–42.

DeBakey, M. E., et al. *The New Living Heart Diet.* New York: Fireside, 1996.

Deckelbaum, R. J., et al. 1999. "Summary of a Scientific Conference on Preventative Nutrition: Pediatrics to Geriatrics." *Circulation.* 100: 450–56.

Demrow, H. S., et al. 1995. "Administration of Wine and Grape Juice Inhibits in Vivo Platelet Activity and Thrombosis in Stenosed Canine Coronary Arteries." *Circulation.* 91: 1182–88.

Dietary Reference Intakes: Calcium, Phosphorus, Magnesium, Vitamin D, and Fluoride. Food and Nutrition Board, Institute of Medicine, prepublication copy, 1997.

Drapkin, R. G., et al. 1995. "Responses to Hypothetical High-Risk Situations: Do They Predict Weight Loss in a Behavioral Treatment Program or the Context of Dietary Lapses?" *Health Psychology.* 14 (5): 427–34.

Ferguson, K. J., and R. L. Spitzer. 1995. "Binge Eating Disorder in a Community-Based Sample of Successful and Unsuccessful Dieters." *International Journal of Eating Disorders.* 18 (2): 167–72.

Fitts, R. H. 1977. "The Effects of Exercise-Training on the Development of Fatigue." *Annals of the New York Academy of Sciences.* 301: 424–30.

Fontaine, K. R., et al. 1998. "Body Mass Index, Smoking, and Mortality Among Older American Women." *Journal of Women's Health.* 7 (10): 1257–61.

Foreyt, J. P., and W. S. C. Poston. 1998. "The Role of the Behavioral Counselor in Obesity Treatment." *Journal of the American Dietetic Association.* 98 (suppl. 2): S27–S30.

Goldberg, A. P. 1989. "Aerobic and Resistive Exercise Modify Risk Factors for Coronary Heart Disease." *Medicine and Science in Sports and Exercise.* 21 (6): 669–77.

Harp, J. B. 1998. "An Assessment of the Efficacy and Safety of Orlistat for the Long-term Management of Obesity." *Journal of Nutrition and Biochemistry.* 9: 516–21.

Hirschmann, J. R., and C. H. Hunter. *Overcoming Overeating.* New York: Fawcett, 1989.

Hollander, P. A., et al. 1998. "Role of Orlistat in the Treatment of Obese Patients with Type 2 Diabetes." *Diabetes Care.* 21 (8): 1288–93.

Kant, A. K., et al. 1995. "Dietary Diversity and Subsequent Cause-Specific Mortality in the NHANES I Epidemiologic Follow-up Study." *Journal of the American College of Nutrition.* 14: 233–38.

———. 1993. "Dietary Diversity and Subsequent Mortality in the First National Health and Nutrition Examination Survey Epidemiologic Follow-up Study." *American Journal of Clinical Nutrition.* 57: 434–40.

Kirk, C. C. 1988. "The Effects of Guided Imagery on Basal Metabolic Rate." *Journal of the Society of Accelerated Learning and Teaching*. 13 (4): 347–61.

Krummel, D. A., and P. M. Kris-Etherton. *Nutrition in Women's Health*. Gaithersburg, Md.: Aspen, 1996, pages 424–25.

Kushi, L. H., et al. 1996. "Dietary Antioxidant Vitamins and Death from Coronary Heart Disease in Postmenopausal Women." *New England Journal of Medicine*. 334: 1156–62.

Lovati, M. R., et al. 1992. "Low-Density Lipoprotein Receptor Activity Is Modulated by Soybean Globulins in Cell Culture." *Journal of Nutrition*. 122: 1971–78.

Mansoor, G. A., et al. 1996. "Determinants of the White-Coat Effect in Hypertensive Subjects." *Journal of Human Hypertension*. 10: 87–92.

Mercer, N. *The M-Fit Grocery Shopping Guide*. Nashville: Favorite Recipes Press, 1995.

National Heart, Lung and Blood Institute in cooperation with the National Institute of Diabetes and Digestive Kidney Diseases. *Clinical Guidelines on the Identification, Evaluation and Treatment of Overweight and Obesity in Adults: The Evidence Report*. September 1998: NIH Publication.

National Heart, Lung and Blood Institute press release: *New High Blood Pressure Guidelines Released by the NHLBI*. November 6, 1997.

National Heart, Lung and Blood Institute publication. *Controlling High Blood Pressure: A Woman's Guide. http://www.nhlbi.nih.gov.*

National Institutes of Health publication. *The Sixth Report of the Joint National Committee on Prevention, Detection, Evaluation and Treatment of High Blood Pressure*. November 1997.

National Task Force on the Prevention and Treatment of Obesity. 1996. "Long-Term Pharmacotherapy in the Management of Obesity." *Journal of the American Medical Association*. 276 (23): 1907–15.

Nordy, A., et al. 1994. "Effects of Dietary Fat Content, Saturated Fatty Acids, and Fish Oil on Eicosanoid Production and Hemotatic Parameters in Normal Men." *Journal of Laboratory and Clinical Medicine*. 123: 914–20.

Pasman, W. J., et al. 1997. "Effect of One Week of Fiber Supplementation on Hunger and Satiety Ratings and Energy Intake." *Appetite*. 29: 77–87.

Pate, R. R., et al. 1995. "Physical Activity and Public Health." *Journal of the American Medical Association*. 273: 404–7.

Pipher, M. *Hunger Pains: The Modern Woman's Tragic Quest for Thinness*. New York: Ballantine, 1995.

Racette S. B., et al. 1995. "Exercise Enhances Dietary Compliance During Moderate Energy Restriction in Obese Women." *American Journal of Clinical Nutrition*. 62: 345–49.

Read, N., et al. 1994. "The Role of the Gut in Regulating Food Intake in Man." *Nutrition Reviews*. 52: 1–10.

Renaud, S., and M. deLorgeril. 1992. "Wine, Alcohol, Platelets, and the French Paradox for Coronary Heart Disease." *Lancet*. 339: 1523–26.

Riggs, B. L., and L. J. Melton. 1992. "The Prevention and Treatment of Osteoporosis." *New England Journal of Medicine*. 327: 620–27.

Riggs, K. M., et al. 1996. "Relations of Vitamin B_{12}, Vitamin B_6, Folate and Homocysteine to Cognitive Performance in the Normative Aging Study." *American Journal of Clinical Nutrition.* 63: 306–14.

Rimm, E. B., et al. 1998. "Folate and Vitamin B_6 from Diet and Supplements in Relation to Risk of Coronary Heart Disease Among Women." *Journal of the American Medical Association.* 279: 359–64.

———. 1993. "Vitamin E Consumption and the Risk of Coronary Heart Disease in Men." *New England Journal of Medicine.* 328: 1450–56.

Roche News Release. "FDA Approves Xenical (Orlistat) for Weight Loss/Maintenance and Reduced Risk of Weight Regain in Obese Patients." Valerie Suga. valeria_a.suga@roche.com

Roche. Xenical (Orlistat) Media Q&A. Valerie Suga. valeria_a.suga@roche.com

Rosengren, A., H. Wedel, and L. Wilhelmsen. 1999. "Body Weight and Weight Gain During Adult Life in Men in Relation to Coronary Heart Disease and Mortality: A Prospective Population Study." *European Heart Journal.* 20 (4): 269–77.

Ruffin, M. T., and M. Cohen. 1994. "Evaluation and Management of Fatigue." *American Family Physician.* (September 1): 625–34.

Sacks, F. M., et al. 1994. "Short Report: The Effect of Fish Oil on Blood Pressure and High-Density Lipoprotein-Cholesterol Levels in Phase I of the Trials of Hypertension Prevention." *Journal of Hypertension.* S23–31.

Sassen, L. M., et al. 1994. "Fish Oil and the Prevention and Regression of Atherosclerosis." *Cardiovascular Drugs and Therapeutics.* 8: 179–91.

Simkin, L. R., and A. M. Gross. 1994. "Assessment of Coping with High-Risk Situations for Exercise Relapse Among Healthy Women." *Health Psychology.* 13 (3): 274–77.

Sjostrom, L., et al. 1998. "Randomized Placebo-Controlled Trial of Orlistat for Weight Loss and Prevention of Weight Regain on Obese Patients." *The Lancet.* 352: 167–72.

Skender, M. L., et al. 1996. "Comparison of Two-Year Weight Loss Trends in Behavioral Treatment of Obesity: Diet, Exercise, and Combination Interventions." *Journal of the American Dietetic Association.* 96 (4): 342–46.

Smallwood, D. M., and J. R. Blaylock. 1994. "Fiber: Not Enough of a Good Thing?" *Food Review* (January–April): 23–29.

"Smarten Up: Certain Foods Help Maintain Brain Power as You Age." *Tufts University Health and Nutrition Letter,* February 1998; 15: 4–5.

Strecher, V. J., et al. 1995. "Goal Setting as a Strategy for Health Behavior Change." *Health Education Quarterly.* 22: 190–200.

"Study Finds Men and Women Overeat for Different Reasons." *Journal of the American Dietetic Association* 1996; 96 (12): 1253.

Tayer, R. E., J. R. Newman, and T. M. McClain. 1994. "Self-Regulation of Mood: Strategies for Changing a Bad Mood, Raising Energy and Reducing Tension." *Journal of Personal and Social Psychology.* 67: 910–25.

Taylor, C. F., J. F. Sallis, and R. Needle. 1985. "The Relation of Physical Activity and Exercise to Mental Health." *Public Health Reports.* 100: 195–202.

The Trials of Hypertension Prevention Collaborative Research Group. 1997.

"Effects of Weight Loss and Sodium Reduction Intervention on Blood Pressure and Hypertension Incidence in Overweight People with High-Normal Blood Pressure." *Archives of Internal Medicine.* 157: 657–67.

Thomas, P. R., ed. *Weighing the Options: Criteria for Evaluating Weight-Management Programs.* Washington, D.C.: National Academy Press, 1995.

Turner, L. W., et al. 1995. "Preventing Relapse in Weight Control: A Discussion of Cognitive and Behavioral Strategies." *Psychology Reports.* 77: 651–56.

Weinberg, R. S. 1994. "Goal Setting and Performance in Sport and Exercise Settings: A Synthesis and Critique." *Medicine and Science in Sports and Exercise.* 26: 469–77.

Index

Recipe entries are in **boldface** type.

abdominal crunches, 176
added fats, 144–45
  fat grams in, 146
  portion sizes for, 143
aerobic exercise, 162
aging, weight maintenance and, 36
alcohol, 73–74
amino acids, 53
animal fats, 57
animal protein, 53, 55
appetite vs. hunger, 216
apple shape body, 37
arachidonic acid, 57
atherosclerosis, 13

bacteria, research on, 19–20
bad food/good food, 49
Baked Apple, 212
balance, in dieting, 48
Banana Almond Oatmeal, 117
Basil-Tossed Rotini Pasta, 211
behavior modification, 27
beverages, hydrating, 73–74, 219–20
bicep curl, 172
Black Bean, Barley, and Leek Soup, 130
Black Bean Salad, 125
blood pressure, high, 13
bloodstream, drug absorption into, 26
blood sugar, 28, 223
body mass index (BMI), 36–37, 38–39
body weight, 31–36
  bone size and, 34–35
  for men, 32–33
  for women, 33–34
bone size, how to determine, 34–35
breakfast:
  recipes for weight loss, 115–19
  recipes for weight maintenance, 199–200
Breakfast Peanut Fruit Salad, 117
breast cancer, 24, 225–26
Breast of Chicken with Braised White Beans and Arugula, 136–37
Broccoli, Mushroom, and Cheese Omelet, 199
Broiled Mandarin Orange Breakfast Sandwich, 200
Buttered Rotini with Chicken Stir-Fry, 204

caffeine, 74
calcium supplement, 182
calories:
from carbohydrates, 18
choosing level of, 70–71
conscientious consumption of, 65
"empty," 51
exercise and burning of, 161
from fat, 18, 55–58
in fat-free food, 50
flexibility in levels of, 71
macronutrients and, 18, 50
minimum intake of, 45
pound equivalent of, 25, 68
from protein, 18, 52
reducing intake of, 26
storage of, 58
three kinds of, 50
weight loss and, 25, 63–64
in weight maintenance, 181
cancer, 14, 24, 225–26
carbohydrates, 50–52
calories and, 18
complex, 51, 52
in daily eating plan, 51–52
low, in diets, 54
simple, 51
Carrot-Broccoli-Lemon Salad, 123
cereal grains, 52
chair squat, 174
Cheese Tomato Omelet, 119
Cheesy Veggie Pile, 122
Chicken and Zucchini Spaghetti, 206
Chicken Stir-Fry, 128
Chicken-Veggie Stir-Fry over Linguine, 133
cholestasis, 41, 221
cholesterol, 56
drugs for lowering of, 222
high levels of, 13
LDL, 57
NCEP and, 46
saturated fat and, 57
Xenical and, 28
ciclosporin, 222
clean plate club, 218–19
clinical trials, 20–23
comfort food, 48–49
comorbid conditions, 37
complementing proteins, 53–54
complex carbohydrates, 51, 52
Confetti Rice Salad, 124
convenience packaged foods, fat in, 145
cooking, low-fat techniques for, 152–53

coronary artery disease, 13
Coumadin, 15, 222–23
counselors, help from, 219
Creamed Chicken on Toast, 132
**Creamy Breakfast Barley with Bananas and
    Dried Cranberries, 200**
Crohn's disease, 16, 41
cross-training, 166–67
cyclosporine (Ciclosporin, Cyclosporin A,
    Sandimmune), 222

dairy foods, fat in, 145, 147
depression, 14
desserts:
    recipes for weight loss, 138–40
    recipes for weight maintenance, 212
diabetes mellitus, 13, 28, 223
diary, food, 143–44, 219
    worksheet for dieting, 144
    worksheet for weight maintenance, 214
diet and exercise program, overview, 43–
    44
dieting, 47–68
    balance in, 48
    calories in, 50, 70–71
    carbohydrates in, 50–52
    comfort foods and, 48–49
    eating out and, 154–55
    fat in, 55–58
    fiber in, 71–72
    food and psychology, 48–49
    good food/bad food in, 49
    high-protein/low carbohydrate, 54
    keeping records in, 143–44, 219
    micronutrients and, 58–62
    monitoring fat in, 144–50
    plateaus in, 66
    protein in, 52–55
    snacks in, 72–73
    understanding food in, 49–62
    water intake in, 73–74, 219–20
    weight goal in, 69–70
    for weight maintenance, 181–82
    without Xenical, 65–67
    with Xenical, 42–43, 67–68
    yo-yo, 157
dining out, 154–55, 224
dinner:
    recipes for weight loss, 126–37
    recipes for weight maintenance,
        204–11
disaccharides, 50–51
doctor:
    advice on exercise from, 159
    issues to discuss with, 41
drinks, hydrating, 73–74, 219–20
drug interactions, 222–23

Easy Garbanzo-Sunflower Salad, 203
eating out, 154–55, 224
essential fatty acids, 57
exercise, 156–78
    abdominal crunches, 176
    aerobic, 162
    bicep curl, 172
    burning calories in, 161
    chair squat, 174
    chart MWF, 173
    chart TTS, 177
    choosing of, 160
    cross-training, 166–67
    diet and, 44
    equipment for, 160
    how much, 161–62
    non-weight-loss benefits of, 157–58
    physician's advice on, 159
    reverse fly, 170
    seated lower leg lift, 176
    single arm row, 170
    starting slowly in, 159
    target heart rate in, 162
    thigh lifts, 175
    top ten for burning fat, 163
    tricep press, 171
    variety in, 160
    walking program, 164–66
    wall push-up, 169
    weight loss and, 156–57
    weight training, 167–78

fat, body, exercises for burning of,
    163
fat, dietary, 55–58
    absorption of, 24–25
    added, 144–45
    added, portion sizes for, 143
    of animal origin, 57
    calories from, 18, 55–58
    daily intake of, 45, 46, 57
    fighting temptation from, 155
    lipids and, 56
    monitoring of, 144–50
    monounsaturated, 56–57
    necessary, 57–58
    of plant origin, 57
    polyunsaturated, 56–57
    saturated, 56–57
    targeting of, 18
    Xenical and, 26–27, 224
fat-free food, 50
fat-soluble vitamins, 224–25
fatty acids:
    essential, 57
    omega-3, 55
Favorite Tuna Pasta Salad, 201

FDA (Food and Drug Administration, U.S.):
    Roche application to, 23–24, 226
    Xenical approved by, 24, 226
fecal urgency, 27
Feta Cheese and Spinach Pizza, 207
fiber, 71–72, 182
fish, omega-3 fatty acids in, 55
fluids, hydrating, 73–74, 219–20
food:
    balance in, 48
    calories in, 50
    carbohydrates in, 50–52
    comfort, 48–49
    control over intake of, 64–65
    fat-free, 50
    fat in, 55–58
    fiber in, 71–72
    good/bad, 49
    macronutrients in, 18, 50
    micronutrients in, 58–62
    negligible fat grams in, 149–50
    portion sizes of, 77–78, 142–43
    protein in, 52–55
    psychology and, 48–49
    stress eating, 217–18
    as tranquilizer, 216
    understanding, 49–62
    volume of, 18
food diary, 143–44, 219
    worksheet for dieting, 144
    worksheet for weight maintenance,
        214
forgiveness, 218
frame size, how to determine, 34–35
**Fresh Garden Salad with Balsamic
    Vinaigrette, 120**
frozen dinners, fat in, 145
fructose, 50
fruit, 52
    portion sizes, 142

galactose, 50
gallstones, 14
gastrointestinal problems, 15–16, 27, 41, 155,
    224
glucose, 50, 223
goal weight, choosing of, 69–70, 217
good food/bad food, 49
grain-based foods, fat in, 145–46, 149
grain food:
    portion sizes, 142
    vegetables, 52
grams, 18
green and leafy vegetables, 52
Green Pepper Omelet, 117
Grilled Asparagus and Leeks, 134
Grilled Vegetable Medley, 126

Ham Sandwich on Rye, 121
heart failure, congestive, 13
heart rate, target, 162
Hearty Chicken Tabbouleh Salad, 130–31
Hearty Vegetable Medley Soup, 206
**Herb-Seared Day Boat Cod with Fresh Stewed
    Tomatoes, 135–36**
Hoffmann-La Roche:
    breast cancer research by, 24, 225–26
    FDA application from, 23–24, 226
    research originated in, 17–20
hormones, 56
hunger vs. appetite, 216
hunger vs. thirst, 220
hydration, 73–74, 219–20
hypoglycemia, 223

inner thigh lift, 175
insulin:
    blood sugar and, 28
    protein and, 54
insulin sensitivity, increasing of, 28
intestinal tract:
    excess fat dumped into, 42–43
    fat absorbed in, 24–25
iron, supplemental, 182
Italian Chicken and Rice, 204–5
Italian Sub, 203

Jenny Craig diet program, 44, 45–46
**Juicy Grilled Hamburger with Vidalia Onion
    on Whole Wheat Bun, 128**

kidney stones, 223
Kris's Split Pea Soup, 126

lactation, Xenical and, 41
LDL cholesterol, 57
**Lean Turkey Sandwich on Whole Wheat,
    120**
leg lift, 176
legumes, 52
**Lemon, Basil, and Ginger Tofu Stir-Fry with
    Spinach Rotini, 127–28**
linoleic acid, 57
linolenic acid, 57
lipase inhibitors:
    action of, 17, 18, 24
    testing of, 18–19
lipases, pancreatic, 18, 25
lipids, 56
lipstatin, identification of, 19
liquids, intake of, 73–74, 219–20
liver, cholesterol and, 57
lunch:
    recipes for weight loss, 119–26
    recipes for weight maintenance, 201–3

macronutrients, 18, 50
maintenance program, *see* weight maintenance
malabsorption, chronic, 15, 41
Mandarin Orange Broil, 122
meatless meals, 55
meats, fat grams in, 148
men, desirable weights for, 32–33
menus, 69–114
    creating your own, 141–53
    food diary and, 143–44, 219
    generic prototype for, 141–42
    how to use, 75–77
    monitoring fat in, 144–50
    planning for, 219
    portion sizes in, 77–78
    Week One, 78–86
    Week Two, 87–114
    Week Three, 96–105
    Week Four, 106–114
    weight maintenance, 183–99
metabolism, exercise and, 157
micronutrients, 58–62
midsection circumference, 37
minerals, supplemental, 58–62
Moistest Pumpkin Muffins, The, 118
monosaccharides, 50, 51
monounsaturated fats, 56–57

NCEP (National Cholesterol Education Program), 46
nursing mothers, Xenical and, 41
nuts, fat in, 145, 149

Oatmeal with Apple and Brown Sugar, 116
obesity, official medical criteria for, 22
Old-Fashioned Apple and Fresh Raspberry Cobbler, 140
omega-3 fatty acids, 55
One Pot Chili, 205
orlistat, 17, 19
    see also Xenical
osteoarthritis, 14
outer thigh lift, 175
overeating moment, freezing of, 218
overweight:
    health concerns and, 13–14
    problems of, 11–16
    solution for, 14–16

packaged foods, convenience, 145
pancreas, action of, 25
pancreatic lipases, 18, 25
pantry, low-fat, 150–52
Parslied Broccoli and Carrots, 209
Parsnip Whipped Potatoes, 133–34

Peach Creamsicle Sundae with Marion Blackberry Fruit Perfect, 139
Peanut Butter and Banana Breakfast Smoothie, 115
pear shape body, 37
Penne with Grilled Chicken and Forest Mushrooms, 137
peptides, 53
physician:
    advice on exercise from, 159
    issues to discuss with, 41
Pita Pocket Turkey Sandwich, 202
Pita Stuffed with Egg, Cheese, and Bacon, 119
Pita Stuffed with Peanut Butter and Banana, 125
plant sources of fat, 57
plant sources of protein, 53, 55
plateaus, in dieting, 66
polysaccharides, 51
polyunsaturated fats, 56–57
Pondimin, 26
Pork and Sweet Potatoes in a Rich Pear Sauce, 211
portions, sizes of, 77–78, 142–43
Portobello Burger, 208
pounds, calorie equivalent of, 25, 68
pravastatin (Pravachol), 15, 222
pregnancy, Xenical and, 41
prolapsing, 215
prostaglandins, 57
protein, 52–55
    amino acids in, 53
    from animal vs. plant sources, 53, 55
    calories and, 18, 52
    complementing, 53–54
    goals for intake of, 55
    portion sizes for, 143
    too much, 54
protein foods, fat in, 145, 147, 148
protein malnutrition, 53
psychology, food and, 48–49

Raspberry Cheesecake, 138
Raspberry-Vanilla Smoothie, 116
recipes, 114–40, 199–212
    breakfast (weight loss), 115–19
    breakfast (weight maintenance), 199–200
    desserts (weight loss), 138–40
    desserts and snacks (weight maintenance), 212
    dinner (weight loss), 126–37
    dinner (weight maintenance), 204–11
    lunch (weight loss), 119–26
    lunch (weight maintenance), 201–3
    see also specific **boldface** *recipe titles*
record-keeping, 143–44, 214, 219
Redux, 26

research:
    bias eliminated in, 21
    clinical trials, 20–23
    compliance in, 22
    for discovery of Xenical, 17–20
    double-blind, 21, 22
    highlights of, 23
    lead-in period of, 22
    placebo-controlled, 21
    publication of results of, 22
    randomized, 21
    results of, 21
    safety and, 22
restaurants, eating in, 154–55, 224
reverse fly, 170
risk factors, 221–22
Roasted Red Pepper, Salmon, and Quinoa
    Salad, 129
Rosemary-Roasted Winter Veggies and
    Chicken, 131
Rotini Chicken Salad with an Asian Peanut
    Sauce, 209

safety concerns, 22, 23–24, 221–27
Salmon Poppyseed Salad, 203
Salsa-Seared Cod, 210
Sandimmune, 222
saturated fats, 56–57
seated lower leg lift, 176
seeds, fat in, 145, 149
serving sizes, 77–78, 142–43
Shrimp Slaw with Jicama, Pineapple and
    Watercress, 135
side effects, 27, 155, 224
simple carbohydrates, 51
single arm row, 170
snacks, 72–73
    low-fat, 45, 144
    in weight maintenance, 181, 212
Sour Cream and Chives Baked Potato, 127
Soy-Orange-Marinated Red Snapper, 132
Spicy Bean Tortilla, 121
Spinach-Lentil Salad, 122
starch, 50
Steamed Veggies with Basil and Olive Oil, 132
sterols, 56
Strawberry-Banana-Kiwi Breakfast Smoothie,
    115
Streptomyces toxitricini bacteria, 19–20
stress eating, 217–18
stroke, 14
sugar, 50
Sweet Pepper Medley, 123

target heart rate, 162
temptation:
    fighting of, 218

giving in to, 155
tetrahydrolipstatin, 19
    see also Xenical
thigh lifts, 175
thirst vs. hunger, 220
Tomato Turkey Stack, 123
torso shapes, 37
Tossed Shrimp Salad, 201
Totally Decadent Banana Chocolate Chip
    Muffins, 212
tricep press, 171
triglycerides, 37, 56
Tuna Fish on Pita, 119
Tuna Tomato Stack, 124
Turkey Burger on Bun with Sliced Vidalia
    Onion, 131

undereating, 218
urinary oxalate, 223

Vegetable Lentil Soup, 202–3
vegetables, 52
    fats from, 57
    portion sizes, 142
    proteins in, 53, 55
vitamins, 58–62
    fat-soluble, 224–25
    K, 222–23
    supplemental, 43, 182

waist circumference, 37
waist-to-hip ratio (WHR), 37
walking, 164–66
walking worksheet, 166
wall push-up, 169
warfarin (Coumadin), 222–23
Warm Pear and Blueberry Granola Crisp with
    Maple Yogurt, 139
water, drinking of, 73–74, 155, 219–20
Watercress Black Bean Salad, 121
waxes, 56
weight:
    bone size and, 34–35
    for men, 32–33
    tracking of, 219
    for women, 33–34
weight control, 12
weight goal, choosing of, 69–70
weight loss:
    behavior modification and, 27
    calorie levels for, 25, 63–64
    exercise and, 156–57
    health benefits of, 27–28
    insulin levels and, 28
    new look at, 11–16
    permanent, 220
    plateaus in, 66

weight loss, *cont.*
    Xenical action and, 24–25
    see also dieting
weight-loss counselors, help from, 219
weight maintenance, 179–220
    aging and, 36
    avoiding weight gain in, 215–20
    clean plate club membership and, 218–19
    counseling for, 219
    diet for, 181–82
    falling backward in, 215–16
    food as tranquilizer in, 216
    forgiveness in, 218
    goals for, 217
    hunger vs. appetite in, 216
    hunger vs. thirst in, 220
    hydration and, 219–20
    keeping records on, 214, 219
    menus, 183–99
    overeating moment frozen in, 218
    planning in, 215, 217, 219
    prolapsing in, 215
    recipes, 199–212
    risky situations and, 217
    stress eating and, 217–18
    temptation avoided in, 218
    tracking weight in, 219
    undereating and, 218
    Xenical and, 180
    on your own, 213–14
weight training, 167–78
Weight Watchers, 44, 45
Western Omelet, 116
WHR (waist-to-hip ratio), 37
Wild Rice with Mushrooms, 210
women, desirable weights for, 33–34
worksheets:
    Calorie Levels for Weight Loss, 63–64
    Cross-Training, 167
    Exercise Chart (Monday, Wednesday, Friday), 173
    Exercise Chart (Tuesday, Thursday, Saturday), 177
    Food Diary (dieting), 144
    Food Diary (weight maintenance), 214

    Is Xenical Right for Me?, 40
    Walking Program, 166
wrist measurement, and frame size, 35

Xenical:
    action of, 24–25
    allergic reactions to, 41
    body mass index and, 36–37, 38–39
    body weight and, 31–36
    breast cancer and, 24, 225–26
    clinical trials of, 20–23
    comorbid conditions and, 37
    diet and exercise program, 43–44
    dieting principles of, 47–68; *see also* dieting
    dieting with, 42–43, 67–68
    dieting without, 65–67
    discussion with doctor about, 41
    drug interactions with, 222–23
    effectiveness of, 15
    fat intake and, 26–27, 224
    FDA approval of, 24, 226
    gastrointestinal problems and, 15–16, 27, 41, 155, 224
    getting optimal effects from, 30–46
    health benefits of, 27–28
    history of, 17–20
    limited action time for, 42, 144, 224
    and other diets, 44–46
    prescribed dose of, 42, 223
    program principles of, 41–42
    proper use of, 42–43
    risk factors for, 221–22
    safety of, 23–24, 221–27
    safe use of, 223–24
    side effects of, 27, 155, 224
    therapeutic window for, 42, 144, 224
    time for taking of, 42, 223–24
    torso shape and, 37
    uniqueness of, 26–27
    vitamin/mineral supplement and, 43, 182
    and weight maintenance, 180
    worksheet (Is Xenical Right for Me?), 40
    worldwide use of, 24

yo-yo dieting, 157